THE COMPLETE
GOOD
ENERGY
COOKBOOK FOR BEGINNERS

Super Easy, 1800 Days of Metabolism-Boosting Recipes + 90-Day Meal Plan to Increase Energy, Support Weight Loss, and Achieve Lasting Wellness

30-Day Good Energy Meal Plan
Printable Shopping List Templates
Quick Reference Cooking Times for Beginners

ORIEL DAVIDSON

Disclaimer

The publisher and author of *The Complete Good Energy Cookbook for Beginners* provide this book and its contents on an "as is" basis, making no claims, guarantees, or warranties regarding the accuracy, reliability, suitability, or completeness of the information. All warranties—express or implied—including, but not limited to, implied warranties of merchantability, fitness for a particular purpose, or non-infringement, are expressly disclaimed.

The information in this book is intended solely for general informational and educational purposes. It does not constitute medical advice and should not be used as a substitute for consultation with a qualified healthcare professional. The recipes, dietary recommendations, and lifestyle tips are designed to promote overall wellness but are not meant to diagnose, treat, or prevent any medical condition. Always consult your doctor or a qualified healthcare provider before significantly changing your diet, exercise routine, or lifestyle, especially if you have specific health concerns.

Individual results may vary, and neither the publisher nor the author can guarantee specific outcomes by applying the information in this book. Testimonials and examples are included for illustrative purposes only and do not guarantee that you will achieve similar results.
By using this book, you agree that the publisher and author shall not be held responsible or liable for any losses, damages, or direct or indirect risks arising from your use or misuse of the content provided.

Table of contents

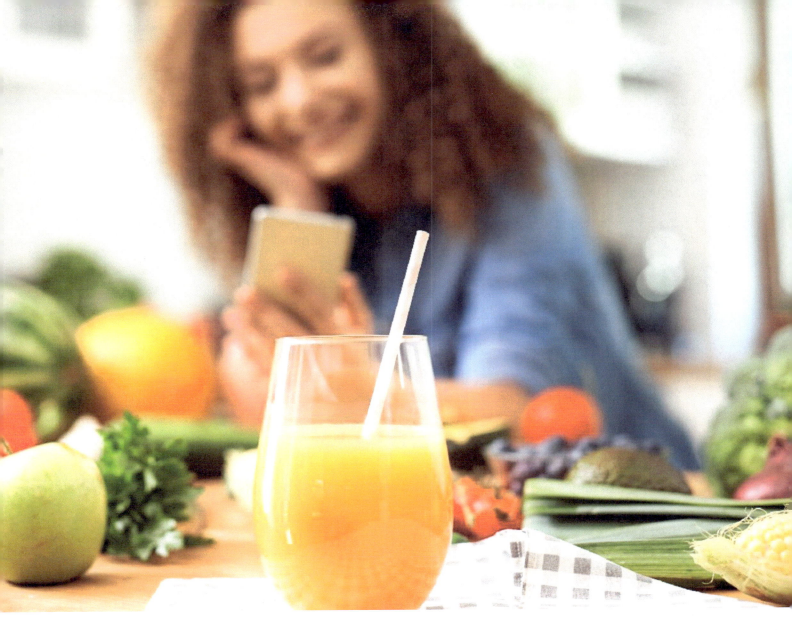

Introduction

Welcome to *The Complete Good Energy Cookbook for Beginners*! This cookbook is more than a collection of recipes—it's your guide to a lifestyle that empowers you to eat healthier, feel more energized, and embrace vibrant well-being. Whether you're new to cooking, exploring more nutritious options, or seeking ways to feel more energized, this book is designed to make your journey simple, enjoyable, and rewarding.

This cookbook, with clear guidance and easy-to-follow recipes, will help you unlock the transformative power of nutrition. Together, we'll explore how the right foods can fuel your body, enhance your mood, and support lasting wellness.

The "Good Energy" Concept

What does it mean to focus on "good energy"? Think of your body as a high-performance engine that thrives on premium fuel. This premium fuel comes from nutrient-dense, whole foods—fresh vegetables, lean proteins, healthy fats, and complex carbohydrates—that provide steady, long-lasting energy.

Unlike crash diets or quick fixes, this approach aligns with your body's natural rhythms, helping you feel energized and focused. A "good energy" diet is about more than just physical vitality—it supports mental clarity, emotional resilience, and a sustainable, healthy lifestyle.

By prioritizing foods that stabilize blood sugar levels, improve metabolism, and nourish your body, you'll not only feel better but also enjoy cooking and eating meals that genuinely satisfy you.

Benefits of an Energy-Focused Diet

1. **Boosting Energy Levels Naturally**
   Say goodbye to energy crashes and afternoon slumps. You can maintain steady energy throughout the day by eating balanced meals that include proteins, healthy fats, and complex carbs.

2. **Improved Digestion**
   Whole, nutrient-dense foods support gut health and make digestion smoother and more efficient.

3. **Weight Management**
   This approach helps you enjoy delicious meals guilt-free while supporting a healthy metabolism.

4. **Mental Clarity**
   Nutrient-rich meals improve focus, concentration, and mood, helping you confidently tackle daily challenges.

5. **Simplicity**
   Energy-focused cooking uses accessible, real ingredients—not complicated meal plans or restrictive diets.

Understanding the Basics of the Good Energy Lifestyle

What Does "Energy-Focused" Eating Mean?

Energy-focused eating isn't about counting calories or chasing quick bursts of energy. It's about giving your body the nutrients it needs to thrive. When you eat whole, nutrient-dense foods, you avoid blood sugar spikes and crashes, feel full longer, and enjoy steady energy that lasts all day.

Why Should Beginners Choose an Energy-Focused Diet?

An energy-focused diet is a simple and practical way for beginners to feel better daily. It offers:

- **Sustained Energy**: Say goodbye to feeling drained by mid-afternoon.
- **Weight Management**: Feel satisfied while supporting a healthy metabolism.
- **Improved Digestion**: Whole foods are easier on your stomach and better for your gut.
- **Mental Clarity**: The right foods can sharpen focus and elevate your mood.

Essential Ingredients for Energy-Focused Cooking

This cookbook highlights easy-to-find ingredients that are perfect for beginners:

- **Whole Grains (Quinoa, Brown Rice, Oats)**: Provide steady energy and fiber.
- **Leafy Greens and Colorful Veggies**: Rich in vitamins and antioxidants.
- **Lean Proteins (Chicken, Fish, Legumes)**: Essential for muscle repair and satiety.
- **Healthy Fats (Avocado, Nuts, Olive Oil)**: Support brain health and provide long-lasting energy.
- **Energizing Snacks (Seeds, Berries, Dark Chocolate)**: Great for a quick boost between meals.

How to Make Energy-Focused Cooking Easy

1. **Meal Prep is Key.**
   Set aside time to chop veggies, cook grains, and portion snacks. This simplifies healthy eating even on your busiest days.
2. **Learn Simple Swaps.**
   Replace refined carbs with whole grains, sugary drinks with herbal tea, and fried snacks with nuts or seeds.
3. **Plan Your Meals.**
   Use the included meal plans to stay organized and make healthy daily choices.
4. **Experiment with Flavors.**
   Try new spices and herbs to make meals exciting without adding unnecessary calories.

Encouragement and Tips for Beginners

Start with Your Favorites
Ease into this lifestyle by starting with meals you already enjoy. For example, try *Zesty Lemon Shrimp Pasta* if you love pasta or *Mediterranean Chickpea Salad* if you like fresh, hearty salads.

Make Cooking Fun
Turn cooking into a joyful activity. Play your favorite music, involve loved ones, and treat it as an act of self-care.

Set Realistic Goals
You don't have to change everything overnight. Focus on small, achievable steps, like trying one new recipe a week or adding an extra serving of veggies.

Celebrate Small Wins
Every healthy choice you make is a victory. Celebrate your progress, no matter how small—it all adds to significant results over time.

Beginner-Friendly Recipe Highlights
This cookbook is designed to make your transition to energy-focused eating seamless. Recipes are:
- **Quick and Simple**: Many take 30 minutes or less.
- **One-Pot or Minimal Cleanup**: Perfect for busy days.
- **Customizable**: Adjust ingredients to your taste and dietary needs.

Examples include:
- *Lemon Dill Baked Cod* – A simple, flavorful dish packed with Omega-3s.
- *Spicy Tuna Poke Bowl* – A fresh, no-cook recipe perfect for beginners.
- *Shrimp Fried Rice* – A quick, satisfying meal for any night of the week.

This isn't just about starting a diet—it's about beginning a lifestyle that prioritizes your health and happiness. There's no rush, and every step forward is progress. Each meal you cook and enjoy is an opportunity to nourish your body, boost your energy, and feel your best.

Welcome to the world of good energy! Let this cookbook guide you as you explore delicious recipes, discover new habits, and create a healthier, more vibrant life.

The Foundations of a Good Energy Diet

The Importance of Balanced Nutrition

- Exploring the principles of a balanced diet for sustained energy.
- Why eating a variety of whole, nutrient-dense foods matters.
- The role of balance in preventing energy crashes and supporting overall health.

Understanding Macronutrients

1. **Carbohydrates: The Body's Primary Energy Source**
   - Simple vs. complex carbohydrates and their effects on energy.
   - Choosing healthy carb sources like whole grains, fruits, and vegetables.
   - The role of fiber in stabilizing blood sugar levels.

2. **Proteins: Building Blocks for Repair and Vitality**
   - The importance of protein for muscle repair, hormones, and enzymes.
   - Best sources of lean protein, including plant-based options.
   - How protein impacts metabolism and satiety.

3. **Fats: Essential for Brain and Hormone Health**
   - Differentiating between healthy fats (unsaturated) and unhealthy fats (trans fats).
   - The role of Omega-3s in reducing inflammation and boosting energy.
   - Foods rich in healthy fats, like avocados, nuts, seeds, and fish.

Understanding Micronutrients

- The importance of vitamins and minerals in optimizing metabolic processes.
- Highlighting key micronutrients for energy, such as B vitamins, magnesium, and iron.
- How to incorporate more micronutrient-rich foods into your meals.

How Nutrition Impacts Energy, Mood, and Focus

- The connection between blood sugar levels and mental clarity.
- How eating patterns can affect your mood and emotional well-being.
- The importance of hydration and its role in energy and focus.
- Tips for timing meals and snacks to maintain energy throughout the day.

Foods to Embrace and Avoid

To create lasting vitality and support your metabolism, focusing on foods that naturally boost energy and avoid those that drain it is essential. Here's how to shape your diet with scientifically-backed recommendations:

Energy-Rich Foods: Fuel Your Body

Incorporating these nutrient-dense foods into your meals will provide sustainable energy, support metabolic function, and promote overall health:

- **Whole Grains:** Quinoa, oats, brown rice, and barley offer complex carbohydrates and fiber for steady energy release.
- **Lean Proteins:** Chicken, turkey, eggs, and plant-based options like tofu and tempeh are essential for muscle repair and metabolic activity.
- **Omega-3-Rich Fish:** Salmon, mackerel, and sardines are rich in essential fatty acids that reduce inflammation and improve brain function.
- **Legumes:** Lentils, chickpeas, and black beans are high in fiber and plant-based protein, keeping you full and energized.
- **Vegetables:** Leafy greens, broccoli, carrots, and bell peppers deliver vitamins, minerals, and antioxidants that combat fatigue.

- **Fruits:** Berries, citrus fruits, apples, and bananas provide natural sugars and nutrients for an instant energy boost.

Foods That Deplete Energy: What to Limit or Avoid

Certain foods can cause energy crashes, disrupt your metabolism, and lead to fatigue. Minimizing these will help you stay energized throughout the day:

- **Processed Foods:** Packaged snacks, fast food, and ready-to-eat meals often contain essential nutrients and unhealthy additives.
- **Added Sugars:** Sweets, sugary drinks, and desserts cause blood sugar spikes followed by crashes, leaving you feeling tired.
- **Trans Fats:** Found in fried foods, margarine, and baked goods, trans fats disrupt metabolic processes and harm cardiovascular health.

Key Takeaway:

Building the foundation of a Good Energy Diet starts with prioritizing nutrient-dense, whole foods while minimizing processed, sugary, and unhealthy options. This approach ensures you're fueling your body for peak vitality and metabolic health.

Kitchen Essentials for Success

To fully embrace the Good Energy Diet, it is essential to set yourself up for success with a well-equipped and organized kitchen. This section highlights the must-have tools and gadgets that streamline meal preparation and make healthy cooking effortless.

1. **Tools for Precision and Portion Control:**
    - **Digital Kitchen Scale**: This measures ingredients accurately and manages portion sizes.
    - **Measuring Cups and Spoons**: Essential for precise measurements of dry and liquid ingredients.

2. **Cutting and Prep Essentials:**
    - **Chef's Knife**: A versatile tool for chopping vegetables, slicing proteins, and more.
    - **Cutting Boards**: Separate boards for produce and proteins to avoid cross-contamination.
    - **Mandoline Slicer**: This is for uniformly slicing vegetables and fruits to reduce prep time.

3. **Cooking Gadgets for Efficiency:**
    - **Blender or Food Processor**: Perfect for smoothies, sauces, and chopping.
    - **Air Fryer**: A healthier alternative to deep-frying, providing crispy textures with minimal oil.
    - **Instant Pot or Slow Cooker**: For cooking hands-free soups, stews, and grains.
    - **Steamer Basket**: This is used to retain nutrients in vegetables and seafood.

4. **Essential Bakeware and Cookware:**
    - **Non-Stick or Cast-Iron Skillets**: For versatile stovetop cooking.
    - **Sheet Pans**: Ideal for roasting vegetables proteins, and making one-pan meals.
    - **Glass or Ceramic Baking Dishes**: For casseroles, baked oats, and desserts.

5. **Storage and Organization Must-Haves:**
    - **Mason Jars or Glass Containers**: These are used to store prepped ingredients and leftovers.
    - **Silicone Bags**: A reusable, eco-friendly option for storing snacks or frozen foods.
    - **Spice Rack or Organizer**: To keep your pantry staples accessible and fresh.

6. **Hydration and Energy Boosting Tools:**
    - **Infuser Water Bottle**: To enhance hydration with fruit and herb flavors.
    - **Juicer**: For fresh, nutrient-packed juices to complement your meals.

Tables for Measurement Conversions

Accurate measurements are crucial for cooking and baking success, especially when following recipes that use different measurement systems. This chapter provides essential conversion tables and tips for using measurement conversions effectively in your kitchen. Whether you're scaling recipes, substituting ingredients, or navigating between metric and imperial systems, these tables will simplify the process.

Metric to Imperial Conversions

Grams ↔ Ounces

Grams (g)	Ounces (oz)
5 g	0.18 oz
10 g	0.35 oz
50 g	1.76 oz
100 g	3.53 oz
250 g	8.82 oz
500 g	17.64 oz
1000 g	35.27 oz

Milliliters ↔ Fluid Ounces

Milliliters (ml)	Fluid Ounces (fl oz)
5 ml	0.17 fl oz
15 ml	0.51 fl oz
30 ml	1.01 fl oz
60 ml	2.03 fl oz
120 ml	4.06 fl oz
240 ml	8.12 fl oz
1000 ml	33.81 fl oz

Kilograms ↔ Pounds

Kilograms (kg)	Pounds (lbs)
0.5 kg	1.10 lbs
1 kg	2.20 lbs
2 kg	4.41 lbs
5 kg	11.02 lbs
10 kg	22.05 lbs

Common Ingredient Conversions

Flour: Cups ↔ Grams

Cups	Grams (g)
1/4 cup	30 g
1/3 cup	40 g
1/2 cup	60 g
1 cup	120 g

Sugar: Cups ↔ Grams

Cups	Grams (g)
1/4 cup	50 g
1/3 cup	67 g
1/2 cup	100 g
1 cup	200 g

Butter: Tablespoons ↔ Grams

Tablespoons	Grams (g)
1 tbsp	14 g
2 tbsp	28 g
4 tbsp	56 g
8 tbsp	113 g

Liquids: Cups ↔ Milliliters

Cups	Milliliters (ml)
1/4 cup	60 ml
1/3 cup	80 ml
1/2 cup	120 ml
1 cup	240 ml

Tips for Using Measurement Conversions in Recipes

Scaling Recipes Up or Down Accurately

1. **Determine the Conversion Factor:** Divide the desired yield by the original yield. For example, if you want to double a recipe for four servings, use a factor of 2.
2. **Apply the Factor to All Ingredients:** Multiply each ingredient's quantity by the conversion factor. Adjust spices and seasonings gradually, as their flavor intensity can vary.
3. **Mind Cooking Times:** Scaled recipes may require adjustments in cooking or baking times. Monitor closely to avoid undercooking or overcooking.

Substituting Ingredients Based on Availability and Preferences

1. **Dry Ingredients:** Use the conversion tables to substitute flour, sugars, and other dry ingredients accurately by weight rather than volume for consistent results.
2. **Liquid Ingredients:** When swapping liquids, match the flavor profile and consistency. For example, milk can often replace cream with slight adjustments to fat content.
3. **Adjust for Regional Ingredients:** Some recipes may call for ingredients unavailable locally. Use conversions to substitute similar items while maintaining balance.

Following these guidelines and utilizing the tables provided, you can cook confidently, regardless of the recipe or measurement system. Let these conversions be your go-to resource for delicious results every time.

Troubleshooting and Tips

Starting and maintaining a good energy diet can be challenging, but with the right strategies and mindset, you can overcome obstacles and stay consistent. This chapter addresses common issues and offers practical solutions and tips to help you adapt recipes, manage your time and budget, and stay motivated on your journey to wellness.

Common Challenges and Solutions

1. **Lack of Time**
   - **Challenge:** Busy schedules can make it hard to prepare meals.
   - **Solution:**
     - **Meal Prep:** Set aside a few hours on the weekend to batch-cook grains, roast vegetables, and portion-out snacks for the week.
     - **Quick Recipes:** Opt for 15- to 30-minute meals like stir-fries, salads, or one-pan dishes.
     - **Use Gadgets:** Tools like slow cookers or pressure cookers save time and simplify cooking.

2. **Budget Constraints**
   - **Challenge:** Eating healthy is perceived as expensive.
   - **Solution:**
     - **Buy in Bulk:** Purchase bulk pantry staples like rice, beans, and nuts to save money.
     - **Seasonal Shopping:** Choose fruits and vegetables in season for better prices and freshness.
     - **Repurpose Ingredients:** To minimize waste, use leftover roasted vegetables in salads or soups.

3. **Picky Eaters or Dietary Preferences**
   - **Challenge:** Accommodating different tastes or food restrictions can be difficult.
   - **Solution:**
     - **Customize Recipes:** Swap proteins, grains, or vegetables in recipes to suit preferences. For example, replace quinoa with brown rice or chicken with tofu.
     - **Allergy-Friendly Alternatives:** Substitute common allergens like nuts with seeds or dairy with plant-based milk.
     - **Family-Friendly Options:** Create build-your-own meals like taco bowls or stir-fries where everyone can choose their ingredients.

4. **Staying Motivated**
   - **Challenge:** Maintaining enthusiasm over time can be tricky.
   - **Solution:**
     - **Set Goals:** Focus on small, achievable goals like trying one new recipe per week.
     - **Track Progress:** Keep a food journal to monitor how your energy levels and mood improve.

- **Involve Others:** Cook with family or friends to make it a fun, shared experience.

Adapting Recipes for Dietary Preferences or Allergies

1. **Plant-Based Alternatives**
   - Replace animal proteins with plant-based options like lentils, chickpeas, tofu, or tempeh.
   - Use nutritional yeast instead of cheese for a savory flavor.

2. **Gluten-Free Adjustments**
   - Swap wheat-based grains with quinoa, rice, or millet.
   - Use gluten-free flour blends for baking or as thickeners.

3. **Dairy-Free Substitutions**
   - Opt for almond, coconut, or oat milk instead of dairy milk.
   - Replace yogurt with unsweetened coconut or almond yogurt.

4. **Nut-Free Options**
   - Use sunflower seeds or pumpkin seeds instead of nuts in recipes.
   - Swap nut-based spreads with sunflower seed butter.

Staying Consistent and Motivated

1. **Plan Ahead:**
   - Schedule time each week to plan meals and grocery shop.
   - Keep your pantry stocked with staples to make meal prep easier.

2. **Stay Flexible:**
   - Don't stress about perfection. If you miss a meal or need to eat out, refocus on your next choice.

3. **Experiment with Variety:**
   - Try new ingredients, spices, or recipes to keep meals exciting.
   - Explore different cuisines to expand your palate.

4. **Celebrate Progress:**
   - Reward yourself for sticking to the plan, whether it's a new kitchen gadget or a relaxing evening off.

Tips for Meal Prep and Consistency

1. **Batch Cooking:**
   - Prepare a big batch of grains, roast several trays of vegetables, or make soups that can be refrigerated or frozen for later use.

2. **Prep Snacks:**
   - Portion nuts, cut vegetables, or prepare energy bites for grab-and-go options.

3. **Label and Store:**
   - Use clear containers with labels to keep your fridge and freezer organized.

4. **Simplify Recipes:**
   - Choose meals with minimal ingredients and easy preparation steps during busy weeks.

Ready to dive into energizing, metabolism-boosting recipes? Let's get started!

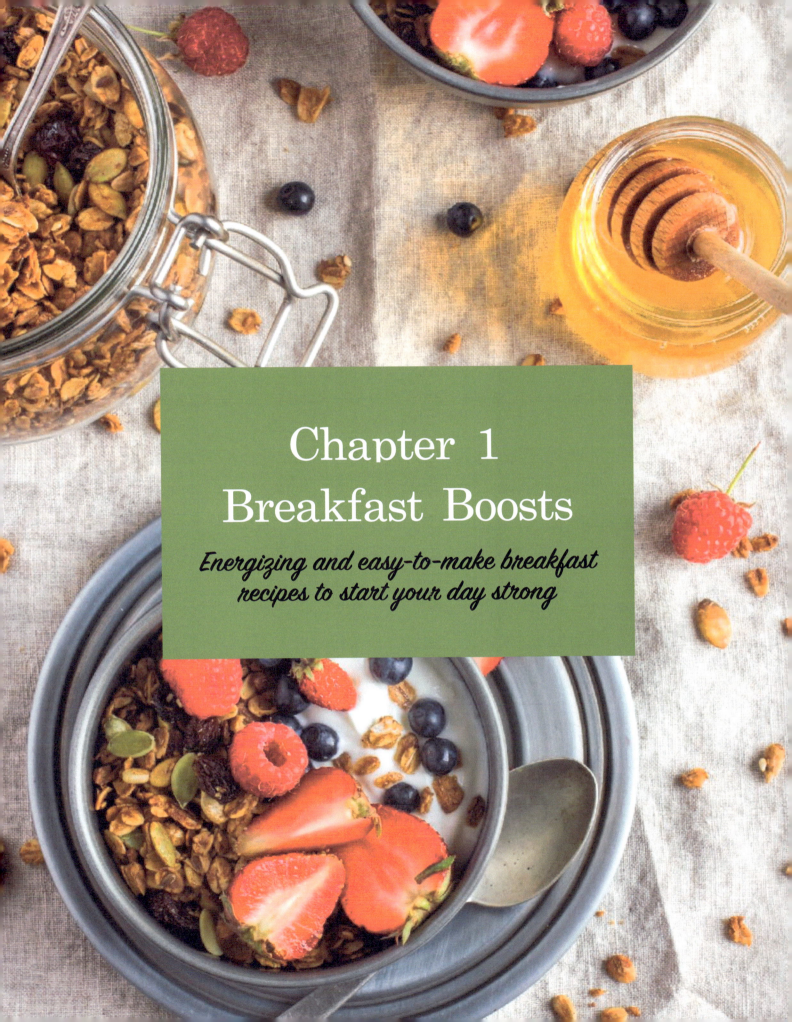

Chapter 1
Breakfast Boosts

*Energizing and easy-to-make breakfast
recipes to start your day strong*

Berry Bliss Overnight Oats with Almond Butter

Yield: 2 servings | Prep time: 10 minutes | Cook time: 0 minutes

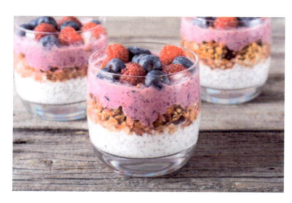

Ingredients:

- 120 g rolled oats
- 250 ml unsweetened almond milk
- 100 g mixed fresh berries (blueberries, raspberries, strawberries)
- 2 tbsp almond butter
- 1 tbsp chia seeds
- 1 tbsp maple syrup (optional)
- 1 tsp vanilla extract

Instructions:

1. Combine rolled oats, almond milk, chia seeds, and vanilla extract in a jar or bowl. Stir well.
2. Add a layer of mixed berries and drizzle almond butter on top.
3. Cover and refrigerate overnight.
4. In the morning, stir it, add more berries if desired, and enjoy.

Nutritional information: 280 calories, 8 g protein, 34 g carbohydrates, 12 g fat, 8 g fiber, 0 mg cholesterol, 75 mg sodium, 250 mg potassium.

Power-Up Green Smoothie with Spinach and Mango

Yield: 2 servings | Prep time: 5 minutes | Cook time: 0 minutes

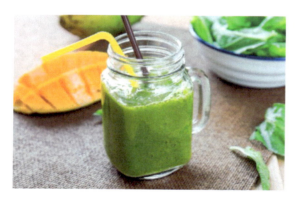

Ingredients:

- 100 g fresh spinach
- 150 g frozen mango chunks
- 1 banana
- 250 ml coconut water
- 1 tbsp chia seeds
- Juice of 1 lime

Instructions:

1. Add spinach, mango, banana, coconut water, chia seeds, and lime juice to a blender.
2. Blend until smooth. Serve immediately.

Nutritional information: 190 calories, 3 g protein, 43 g carbohydrates, 2 g fat, 5 g fiber, 0 mg cholesterol, 45 mg sodium, 400 mg potassium.

Protein-Packed Breakfast Burrito with Black Beans

Yield: 4 servings | Prep time: 10 minutes | Cook time: 10 minutes

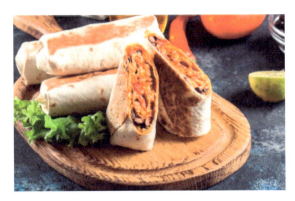

Ingredients:

- 4 whole-grain tortillas (20 cm each)
- 4 large eggs
- 100 g black beans, cooked
- 100 g shredded cheddar cheese
- 1 avocado, sliced
- 1 small tomato, diced
- 1 tbsp olive oil
- 1 tsp ground cumin
- Salt and pepper to taste

Instructions:

1. In a pan, heat olive oil over medium heat. Add eggs, season with cumin, salt, and pepper, and scramble until cooked.
2. Warm tortillas in a dry pan or microwave.
3. Assemble burritos by layering scrambled eggs, black beans, cheese, avocado slices, and diced tomato.
4. Roll tightly and serve warm.

Nutritional information: 340 calories, 15 g protein, 29 g carbohydrates, 18 g fat, 6 g fiber, 180 mg cholesterol, 370 mg sodium, 500 mg potassium.

Fluffy Egg White and Veggie Omelette

Yield: 2 servings | Prep time: 10 minutes | Cook time: 5 minutes

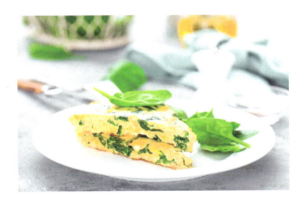

Ingredients:

- 6 egg whites
- 50 g baby spinach
- 50 g cherry tomatoes, halved
- 30 g feta cheese, crumbled
- 1 tbsp olive oil
- Salt and pepper to taste

Instructions:

1. Heat olive oil in a non-stick pan over medium heat.
2. Add spinach and cherry tomatoes, sauté for 2 minutes.
3. Pour egg whites, season with salt and pepper, and cook until set.
4. Sprinkle feta cheese on top, fold, and serve.

Nutritional information: 150 calories, 14 g protein, 3 g carbohydrates, 9 g fat, 2 g fiber, 5 mg cholesterol, 300 mg sodium, 350 mg potassium.

Warm Apple-Cinnamon Quinoa Bowl

Yield: 3 servings | Prep time: 10 minutes | Cook time: 20 minutes

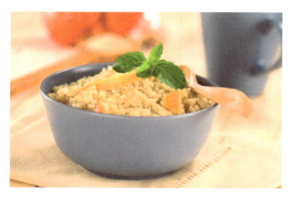

Ingredients:

- 150 g quinoa
- 300 ml water
- 1 medium apple, diced
- 250 ml almond milk
- 1 tbsp maple syrup
- 1 tsp ground cinnamon
- 1 tbsp chopped walnuts

Instructions:

1. Rinse quinoa and cook in water until tender (about 15 minutes).
2. Combine cooked quinoa, almond milk, apple, cinnamon, and maple syrup in a saucepan. Simmer for 5 minutes.
3. Serve warm, topped with walnuts.

Nutritional information: 230 calories, 6 g protein, 39 g carbohydrates, 5 g fat, 4 g fiber, 0 mg cholesterol, 10 mg sodium, 180 mg potassium.

Avocado and Smoked Salmon Toast

Yield: 2 servings | Prep time: 5 minutes | Cook time: 0 minutes

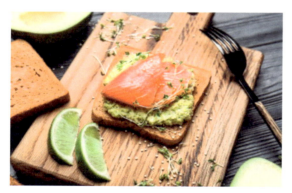

Ingredients:

- 2 slices whole-grain bread
- 1 avocado, mashed
- 60 g smoked salmon
- Juice of 1 lemon
- Fresh dill for garnish

Instructions:

1. Toast bread slices.
2. Spread mashed avocado on each slice.
3. Top with smoked salmon, drizzle with lemon juice and garnish with dill.

Nutritional information: 280 calories, 12 g protein, 20 g carbohydrates, 18 g fat, 6 g fiber, 20 mg cholesterol, 300 mg sodium, 400 mg potassium.

Energy-Boosting Peanut Butter Banana Smoothie

Yield: 2 servings | Prep time: 5 minutes | Cook time: 0 minutes

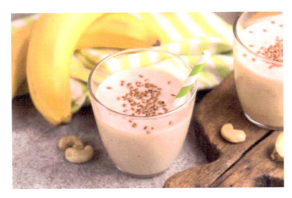

Ingredients:
- 2 bananas
- 250 ml almond milk
- 2 tbsp natural peanut butter
- 1 tsp honey
- 1 tbsp flaxseed
- Ice cubes

Instructions:
1. Combine all ingredients in a blender.
2. Blend until smooth and serve immediately.

Nutritional information: 310 calories, 8 g protein, 40 g carbohydrates, 12 g fat, 6 g fiber, 0 mg cholesterol, 80 mg sodium, 450 mg potassium.

Chia Seed Pudding with Fresh Berries

Yield: 3 servings | Prep time: 10 minutes | Cook time: 0 minutes

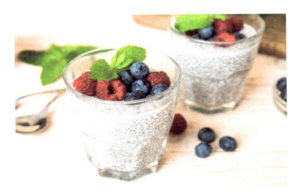

Ingredients:
- 60 g chia seeds
- 300 ml almond milk
- 1 tbsp maple syrup
- 100 g mixed fresh berries

Instructions:
1. Mix chia seeds, almond milk, and maple syrup in a bowl. Stir well.
2. Refrigerate for at least 4 hours or overnight.
3. Serve topped with fresh berries.

Nutritional information: 200 calories, 6 g protein, 18 g carbohydrates, 9 g fat, 8 g fiber, 0 mg cholesterol, 60 mg sodium, 200 mg potassium

Sweet Potato and Chickpea Breakfast Bowl

Yield: 4 servings | Prep time: 10 minutes | Cook time: 25 minutes

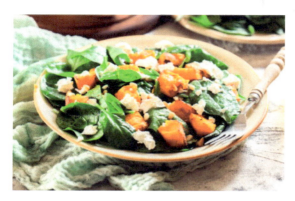

Ingredients:
- 2 medium sweet potatoes, diced
- 200 g cooked chickpeas
- 1 tbsp olive oil
- 1 tsp smoked paprika
- 100 g baby spinach
- 50 g crumbled feta cheese
- Salt and pepper to taste

Instructions:
1. Preheat oven to 200°C.
2. Toss sweet potatoes with olive oil, smoked paprika, salt, and pepper. Roast for 20 minutes.
3. Combine roasted sweet potatoes, chickpeas, spinach, and feta cheese in a bowl. Serve warm.

Nutritional information: 290 calories, 9 g protein, 35 g carbohydrates, 10 g fat, 8 g fiber, 10 mg cholesterol, 200 mg sodium, 500 mg potassium.

Zucchini and Feta Muffins for On-the-Go Energy

Yield: 6 servings | Prep time: 10 minutes | Cook time: 25 minutes

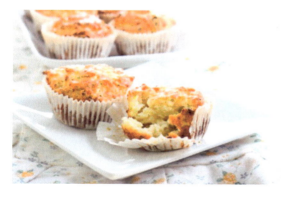

Ingredients:
- 200 g grated zucchini
- 100 g feta cheese, crumbled
- 100 g whole-grain flour
- 2 large eggs
- 1 tsp baking powder
- 50 ml olive oil
- Salt and pepper to taste

Instructions:
1. Preheat oven to 180°C and line a muffin tin with liners.
2. Mix zucchini, feta cheese, eggs, olive oil, baking powder, and flour until combined.
3. Spoon mixture into muffin tins and bake for 25 minutes.
4. Let cool before serving.

Nutritional information: 180 calories, 7 g protein, 12 g carbohydrates, 12 g fat, 2 g fiber, 45 mg cholesterol, 200 mg sodium, 250 mg potassium.

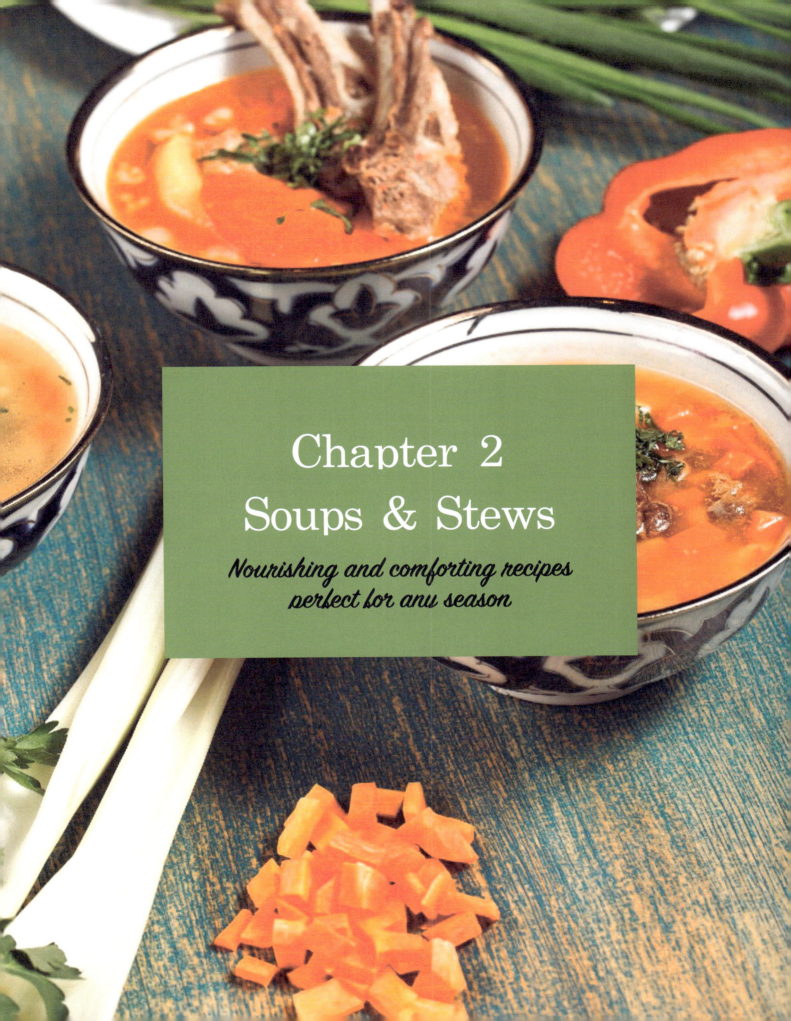

Chapter 2
Soups & Stews

*Nourishing and comforting recipes
perfect for any season*

Creamy Roasted Tomato Basil Soup

Yield: 4 servings | Prep time: 15 minutes | Cook time: 30 minutes

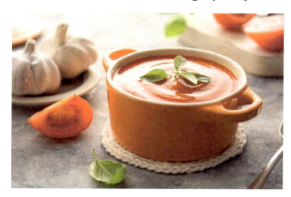

Ingredients:
- 1 kg ripe tomatoes, halved
- 2 medium onions, diced (200 g)
- 4 cloves garlic, minced
- 2 tbsp olive oil
- 500 ml vegetable stock
- 150 ml heavy cream
- 1 handful fresh basil leaves
- 1 tsp salt
- 1/2 tsp black pepper

Instructions:
1. Preheat oven to 200°C. Place halved tomatoes on a baking sheet, drizzle with 1 tbsp olive oil, and roast for 20 minutes.
2. Heat 1 tbsp olive oil in a large pot over medium heat. Sauté onions and garlic until soft.
3. Add roasted tomatoes, vegetable stock, salt, and pepper to the pot. Simmer for 10 minutes.
4. Blend the soup until smooth using an immersion blender. Stir in heavy cream and basil leaves.
5. Serve hot, garnished with additional basil leaves.

Nutritional information: 250 calories, 4 g protein, 18 g carbohydrates, 18 g fat, 3 g fiber, 25 mg cholesterol, 500 mg sodium, 450 mg potassium.

Hearty Lentil and Vegetable Stew

Yield: 6 servings | Prep time: 20 minutes | Cook time: 40 minutes

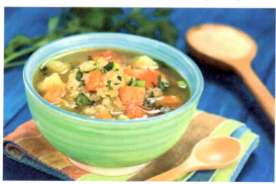

Ingredients:
- 200 g cooked chicken breast, shredded
- 100 g quinoa, rinsed
- 1 L chicken stock
- 2 medium carrots, diced (200 g)
- 2 celery stalks, diced (150 g)
- 1 medium onion, diced (100 g)
- 1 tbsp olive oil
- 1/2 tsp dried thyme
- 1/2 tsp dried parsley
- 1/2 tsp salt
- 1/4 tsp black pepper

Instructions:
1. Heat olive oil in a large pot over medium heat. Sauté onion, carrots, and celery until softened.
2. Add chicken stock, quinoa, thyme, and parsley. Bring to a boil.
3. Reduce heat to low and simmer for 20 minutes until quinoa is cooked.
4. Stir in shredded chicken, salt, and pepper. Heat through for 5 minutes.
5. Serve warm, garnished with fresh parsley if desired.

Nutritional information: 240 calories, 18 g protein, 20 g carbohydrates, 7 g fat, 4 g fiber, 40 mg cholesterol, 500 mg sodium, 450 mg potassium.

Golden Turmeric and Ginger Carrot Soup

Yield: 4 servings | Prep time: 15 minutes | Cook time: 25 minutes

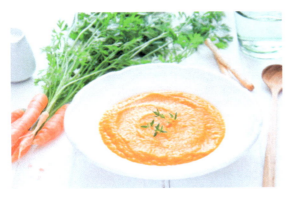

Ingredients:
- 600 g carrots, peeled and sliced
- 1 medium onion, diced (100 g)
- 2 cloves garlic, minced
- 1 tbsp fresh ginger, grated
- 1 tsp ground turmeric
- 750 ml vegetable stock
- 1 tbsp olive oil
- 150 ml coconut milk
- 1/2 tsp salt
- 1/4 tsp black pepper

Instructions:
1. Heat olive oil in a large pot over medium heat. Sauté onion, garlic, and ginger until fragrant.
2. Add carrots, turmeric, and vegetable stock. Simmer for 20 minutes until carrots are tender.
3. Blend the soup until smooth using an immersion blender. Stir in coconut milk, salt, and pepper.
4. Serve warm, garnished with a swirl of coconut milk.

Nutritional information: 180 calories, 3 g protein, 20 g carbohydrates, 10 g fat, 4 g fiber, 0 mg cholesterol, 350 mg sodium, 500 mg potassium.

Classic Chicken and Quinoa Soup

Yield: 4 servings | Prep time: 15 minutes | Cook time: 30 minutes

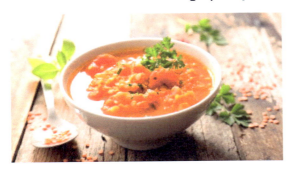

Ingredients:
- 250 g dried lentils, rinsed
- 1.5 L vegetable stock
- 2 medium carrots, diced (200 g)
- 2 celery stalks, diced (150 g)
- 1 medium onion, diced (100 g)
- 2 medium potatoes, cubed (300 g)
- 2 tbsp olive oil
- 1 tsp smoked paprika
- 1 tsp ground cumin
- 1/2 tsp salt
- 1/4 tsp black pepper

Instructions:
1. Heat olive oil in a large pot over medium heat. Sauté onion, carrot, and celery until soft.
2. Add potatoes, lentils, and spices. Stir to coat.
3. Pour in vegetable stock. Bring to a boil, then reduce heat and simmer for 30-40 minutes, until lentils and potatoes are tender.
4. Adjust seasoning to taste and serve warm.

Nutritional information: 290 calories, 12 g protein, 45 g carbohydrates, 6 g fat, 12 g fiber, 0 mg cholesterol, 700 mg sodium, 600 mg potassium.

Savory Sweet Potato and Coconut Curry Stew

Yield: 4 servings | Prep time: 20 minutes | Cook time: 30 minutes

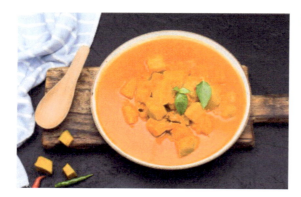

Ingredients:
- 500 g sweet potatoes, peeled and cubed
- 1 medium onion, diced (100 g)
- 2 cloves garlic, minced
- 1 tbsp fresh ginger, grated
- 400 ml canned coconut milk
- 500 ml vegetable stock
- 2 tbsp red curry paste
- 1 tbsp olive oil
- 1 tsp ground coriander
- 1 tsp ground cumin
- 1/2 tsp salt
- 1/4 tsp black pepper

Instructions:
1. Heat olive oil in a large pot over medium heat. Sauté onion, garlic, and ginger until fragrant.
2. Add sweet potatoes, curry paste, coriander, and cumin. Stir to coat.
3. Pour in coconut milk and vegetable stock. Simmer for 25-30 minutes until sweet potatoes are tender.
4. Adjust seasoning to taste. Serve warm, garnished with fresh cilantro if desired.

Nutritional information: 300 calories, 4 g protein, 35 g carbohydrates, 16 g fat, 6 g fiber, 0 mg cholesterol, 500 mg sodium, 600 mg potassium.

Mediterranean Chickpea and Spinach Soup

Yield: 4 servings | Prep time: 15 minutes | Cook time: 25 minutes

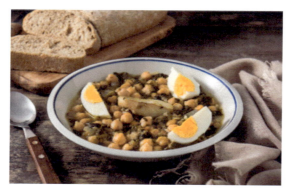

Ingredients:
- 1 can (400 g) chickpeas, drained and rinsed
- 150 g fresh spinach
- 1 medium onion, diced (100 g)
- 2 cloves garlic, minced
- 1 L vegetable stock
- 2 tbsp olive oil
- 1 tsp dried oregano
- 1/2 tsp smoked paprika
- 1/2 tsp salt
- 1/4 tsp black pepper

Instructions:
1. Heat olive oil in a large pot over medium heat. Sauté onion and garlic until fragrant.
2. Add chickpeas, vegetable stock, oregano, and smoked paprika. Simmer for 15 minutes.
3. Stir in fresh spinach and cook for 5 minutes until wilted.
4. Adjust seasoning to taste and serve warm.

Nutritional information: 220 calories, 8 g protein, 24 g carbohydrates, 10 g fat, 6 g fiber, 0 mg cholesterol, 450 mg sodium, 500 mg potassium.

Slow-Cooked Beef and Root Vegetable Stew

Yield: 6 servings | Prep time: 20 minutes | Cook time: 2 hours

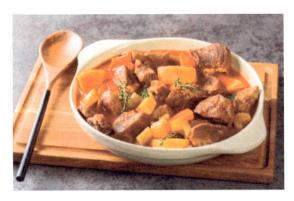

Ingredients:
- 500 g beef chuck, cubed
- 2 medium potatoes, cubed (300 g)
- 2 medium carrots, diced (200 g)
- 2 celery stalks, diced (150 g)
- 1 medium onion, diced (100 g)
- 1 L beef stock
- 2 tbsp tomato paste
- 2 tbsp olive oil
- 1 tsp dried rosemary
- 1 tsp dried thyme
- 1/2 tsp salt
- 1/4 tsp black pepper

Instructions:
1. Heat olive oil in a large pot. Brown beef cubes on all sides, then remove from the pot.
2. Sauté onion, carrots, celery, and potatoes in the same pot until softened.
3. Add beef back to the pot with tomato paste, rosemary, thyme, salt, and pepper. Stir to combine.
4. Pour in beef stock. Cover and simmer on low heat for 2 hours until beef is tender.
5. Serve warm, garnished with fresh parsley.

Nutritional information: 320 calories, 22 g protein, 18 g carbohydrates, 15 g fat, 3 g fiber, 60 mg cholesterol, 600 mg sodium, 700 mg potassium.

Zesty Lemon and Dill Fish Soup

Yield: 4 servings | Prep time: 15 minutes | Cook time: 25 minutes

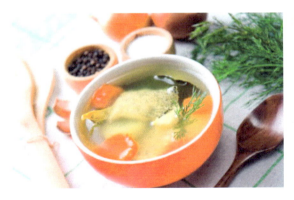

Ingredients:
- 300 g white fish fillets (e.g., cod), cubed
- 1 medium onion, diced (100 g)
- 1 medium carrot, diced (100 g)
- 1 celery stalk, diced (75 g)
- 1 L fish stock
- 1 tbsp olive oil
- 1 lemon, zested and juiced
- 2 tbsp fresh dill, chopped
- 1/2 tsp salt
- 1/4 tsp black pepper

Instructions:
1. Heat olive oil in a large pot over medium heat. Sauté onion, carrot, and celery until softened.
2. Add fish stock, lemon zest, and juice. Bring to a simmer.
3. Add fish cubes and cook for 10 minutes until the fish is cooked.
4. Stir in fresh dill, salt, and pepper. Serve warm.

Nutritional information: 190 calories, 20 g protein, 8 g carbohydrates, 8 g fat, 2 g fiber, 50 mg cholesterol, 400 mg sodium, 450 mg potassium.

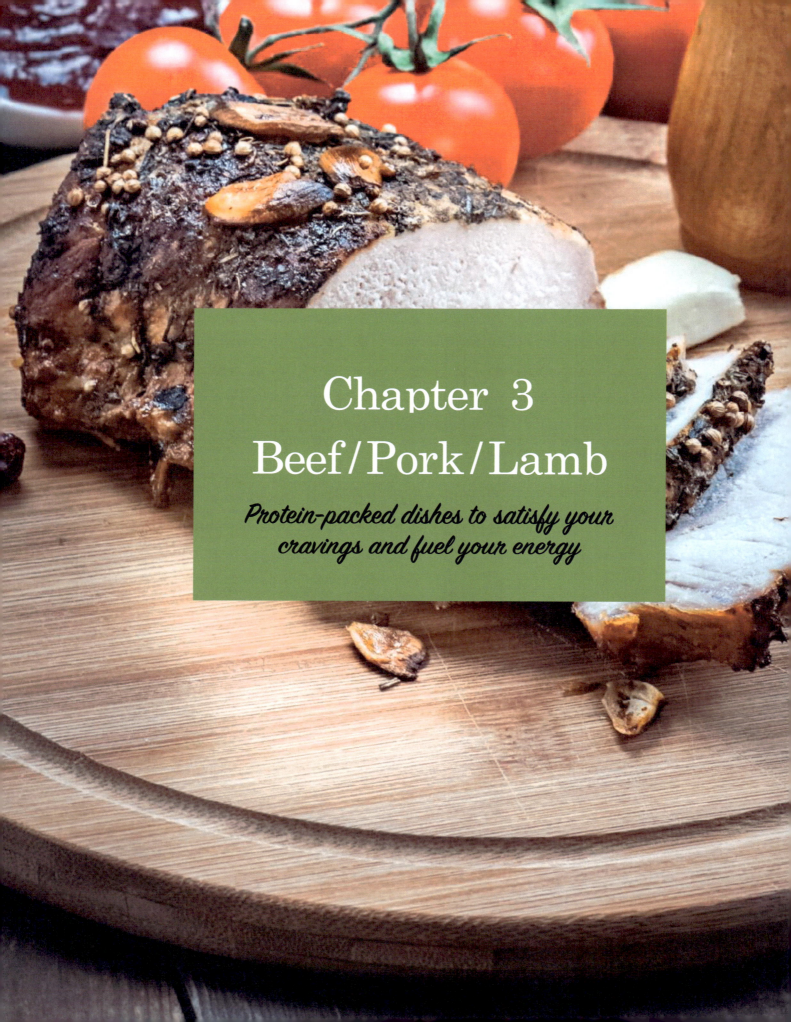

Chapter 3
Beef/Pork/Lamb

Protein-packed dishes to satisfy your cravings and fuel your energy

Savory Herb-Crusted Beef Tenderloin

Yield: 4 servings | Prep time: 15 minutes | Cook time: 40 minutes

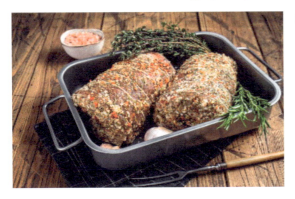

Ingredients:
- 800 g beef tenderloin
- 30 g Dijon mustard
- 60 g breadcrumbs
- 30 g Parmesan cheese, grated
- 2 cloves garlic, minced
- 15 g fresh rosemary, chopped
- 15 g fresh thyme, chopped
- 10 g fresh parsley, chopped
- 30 ml olive oil
- 5 g salt
- 2 g black pepper

Instructions:
1. Preheat the oven to 200°C.
2. Pat the beef tenderloin dry and season with salt and pepper.
3. Spread Dijon mustard evenly over the surface of the beef.
4. Mix breadcrumbs, Parmesan, garlic, rosemary, thyme, parsley, and olive oil in a bowl.
5. Press the herb mixture onto the beef to create an even crust.
6. Place the beef on a baking tray and roast for 30–40 minutes, or until the internal temperature reaches 55°C for medium-rare.
7. Remove from the oven, cover with foil, and let rest for 10 minutes before slicing.

Nutritional information: 375 calories, 37 g protein, 6 g carbohydrates, 24 g fat, 1 g fiber, 95 mg cholesterol, 320 mg sodium, 530 mg potassium.

Quick and Easy Beef Stir-Fry with Vegetables

Yield: 4 servings | Prep time: 10 minutes | Cook time: 15 minutes

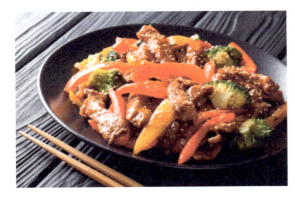

Ingredients:
- 500 g beef sirloin, thinly sliced
- 30 ml soy sauce
- 15 ml oyster sauce
- 10 ml sesame oil
- 5 g cornstarch
- 2 cloves garlic, minced
- 10 g ginger, grated
- 200 g broccoli florets
- 150 g bell peppers, sliced
- 100 g carrots, julienned
- 30 ml vegetable oil

Instructions:
1. Toss beef with soy sauce, oyster sauce, sesame oil, and cornstarch. Set aside for 10 minutes.
2. Heat vegetable oil in a wok or skillet over high heat. Add garlic and ginger; stir-fry for 30 seconds.
3. Add beef and stir-fry until browned, about 3 minutes. Remove and set aside.
4. Add broccoli, bell peppers, and carrots to the wok. Stir-fry for 5 minutes until tender-crisp.
5. Return beef to the wok and toss to combine. Serve immediately.

Nutritional information: 290 calories, 27 g protein, 10 g carbohydrates, 17 g fat, 3 g fiber, 75 mg cholesterol, 420 mg sodium, 470 mg potassium.

Hearty Classic Beef and Barley Stew

Yield: 6 servings | Prep time: 15 minutes | Cook time: 2 hours

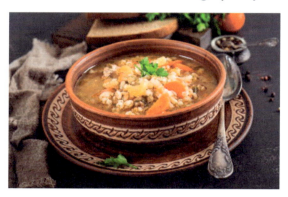

Ingredients:
- 700 g beef chuck, cut into 2.5 cm cubes
- 15 ml olive oil
- 1 onion, diced
- 2 cloves garlic, minced
- 2 carrots, sliced
- 2 celery stalks, sliced
- 200 g pearl barley
- 1.5 L beef stock
- 400 g canned diced tomatoes
- 2 bay leaves
- 5 g fresh thyme
- 10 g salt
- 3 g black pepper

Instructions:
1. Heat olive oil in a large pot over medium-high heat. Brown the beef cubes, then set aside.
2. Add onion, garlic, carrots, and celery to the pot. Sauté until softened, about 5 minutes.
3. Stir in barley, stock, tomatoes, bay leaves, thyme, salt, and pepper. Return beef to the pot.
4. Bring to a boil, then reduce heat to low. Simmer covered for 1.5–2 hours, stirring occasionally.
5. Remove bay leaves before serving.

Nutritional information: 320 calories, 28 g protein, 25 g carbohydrates, 12 g fat, 6 g fiber, 80 mg cholesterol, 650 mg sodium, 620 mg potassium.

Grilled Flank Steak with Chimichurri Sauce

Yield: 4 servings | Prep time: 20 minutes | Cook time: 10 minutes

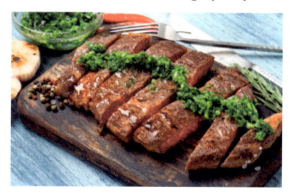

Ingredients:
- 700 g flank steak
- 30 ml olive oil
- 10 g salt
- 3 g black pepper
- 15 g fresh parsley
- 10 g fresh cilantro
- 2 cloves garlic
- 60 ml olive oil (for sauce)
- 30 ml red wine vinegar
- 1 g red pepper flakes

Instructions:
1. Rub steak with olive oil, salt, and pepper. Let it rest at room temperature for 15 minutes.
2. Preheat the grill to high heat. Grill steak for 4–5 minutes per side for medium-rare.
3. To make the chimichurri sauce, combine parsley, cilantro, garlic, olive oil, vinegar, and red pepper flakes in a blender.
4. Let the steak rest for 5 minutes before slicing. Serve with the sauce.

Nutritional information: 365 calories, 31 g protein, 2 g carbohydrates, 26 g fat, 0 g fiber, 85 mg cholesterol, 320 mg sodium, 580 mg potassium.

Slow-cooked beef Ragu over Whole-Wheat Pasta

Yield: 6 servings | Prep time: 15 minutes | Cook time: 6 hours

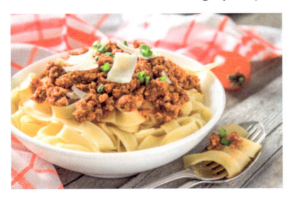

Ingredients:
- 1 kg beef chuck, cut into chunks
- 30 ml olive oil
- 1 onion, diced
- 2 cloves garlic, minced
- 400 g canned crushed tomatoes
- 200 ml red wine
- 15 g tomato paste
- 2 bay leaves
- 5 g fresh rosemary
- 10 g salt
- 300 g whole-wheat pasta

Instructions:
1. Heat olive oil in a skillet. Brown beef on all sides, then transfer to a slow cooker.
2. Add onion and garlic to the skillet; sauté for 3 minutes. Transfer to the slow cooker.
3. Add tomatoes, wine, paste, bay leaves, rosemary, and salt. Cook on low for 6 hours.
4. Cook pasta according to package instructions.
5. Shred the beef with forks and toss with the sauce. Serve over pasta.

Nutritional information: 440 calories, 35 g protein, 35 g carbohydrates, 15 g fat, 7 g fiber, 90 mg cholesterol, 480 mg sodium, 650 mg potassium.

Honey Garlic Glazed Pork Chops

Yield: 4 servings | Prep time: 10 minutes | Cook time: 20 minutes

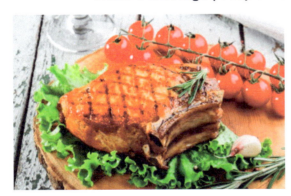

Ingredients:
- 600 g bone-in pork chops
- 30 g honey
- 30 ml soy sauce
- 2 cloves garlic, minced
- 10 g fresh parsley, chopped (optional, for garnish)
- 30 ml olive oil
- 5 g salt
- 2 g black pepper

Instructions:
1. Season pork chops with salt and pepper.
2. Heat olive oil in a skillet over medium-high heat. Sear pork chops for 3–4 minutes per side until golden brown.
3. Reduce heat to medium. Add honey, soy sauce, and garlic to the skillet. Simmer for 5–7 minutes, basting chops with the sauce until it thickens slightly.
4. Garnish with parsley before serving.

Nutritional information: 310 calories, 28 g protein, 10 g carbohydrates, 18 g fat, 0 g fiber, 85 mg cholesterol, 580 mg sodium, 470 mg potassium.

Tender Pulled Pork with Smoky Barbecue Sauce

Yield: 6 servings | Prep time: 15 minutes | Cook time: 6 hours

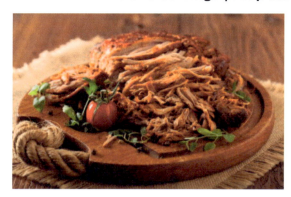

Ingredients:
- 1.2 kg pork shoulder
- 10 g smoked paprika
- 5 g garlic powder
- 5 g onion powder
- 10 g salt
- 3 g black pepper
- 200 g barbecue sauce
- 200 ml chicken stock

Instructions:
1. Rub pork with smoked paprika, garlic powder, onion powder, salt, and pepper.
2. Place pork in a slow cooker. Add chicken stock and barbecue sauce.
3. Cook on low for 6 hours or until tender.
4. Shred the pork with forks and toss with the sauce. Serve on buns or as desired.

Nutritional information: 340 calories, 28 g protein, 12 g carbohydrates, 20 g fat, 0 g fiber, 85 mg cholesterol, 540 mg sodium, 450 mg potassium.

Herbed Pork Tenderloin with Roasted Vegetables

Yield: 4 servings | Prep time: 15 minutes | Cook time: 35 minutes

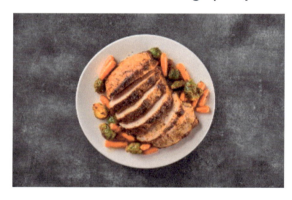

Ingredients:
- 700 g pork tenderloin
- 15 ml olive oil
- 10 g fresh rosemary, chopped
- 5 g fresh thyme, chopped
- 5 g salt
- 2 g black pepper
- 300 g baby carrots
- 200 g Brussels sprouts, halved
- 200 g potatoes, cubed

Instructions:
1. Preheat the oven to 200°C.
2. Rub pork with olive oil, rosemary, thyme, salt, and pepper. Place on a baking sheet.
3. Toss carrots, Brussels sprouts, and potatoes with olive oil, salt, and pepper. Arrange around the pork.
4. Roast for 30–35 minutes or until the pork reaches an internal temperature of 63°C. Let rest for 5 minutes before slicing.

Nutritional information: 320 calories, 30 g protein, 18 g carbohydrates, 12 g fat, 3 g fiber, 80 mg cholesterol, 480 mg sodium, 600 mg potassium.

Sweet and Savory Pork Stir-Fry with Pineapple

Yield: 4 servings | Prep time: 10 minutes | Cook time: 15 minutes

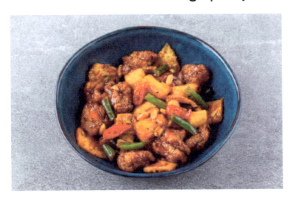

Ingredients:
- 500 g pork loin, thinly sliced
- 200 g pineapple chunks (fresh or canned)
- 30 ml soy sauce
- 15 ml hoisin sauce
- 10 ml sesame oil
- 5 g cornstarch
- 2 cloves garlic, minced
- 150 g bell peppers, sliced
- 100 g snap peas
- 30 ml vegetable oil

Instructions:
1. Toss pork with soy sauce, hoisin sauce, sesame oil, and cornstarch. Set aside for 10 minutes.
2. Heat vegetable oil in a wok over high heat. Stir-fry garlic for 30 seconds.
3. Add pork and cook for 3–4 minutes until browned. Remove and set aside.
4. Stir-fry bell peppers and snap peas for 4 minutes. Add pineapple and return the pork to the wok.
5. Stir to combine and serve immediately.

Nutritional information: 280 calories, 26 g protein, 16 g carbohydrates, 12 g fat, 2 g fiber, 75 mg cholesterol, 520 mg sodium, 430 mg potassium.

Crispy Garlic and Rosemary Pork Cutlets

Yield: 4 servings | Prep time: 15 minutes | Cook time: 20 minutes

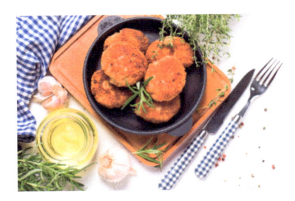

Ingredients:
- 500 g pork cutlets
- 100 g breadcrumbs
- 30 g Parmesan cheese, grated
- 10 g fresh rosemary, chopped
- 2 cloves garlic, minced
- 2 large eggs, beaten
- 50 g all-purpose flour
- 30 ml olive oil
- 5 g salt
- 2 g black pepper

Instructions:
1. Mix breadcrumbs, Parmesan, rosemary, and garlic in a shallow dish.
2. Coat pork cutlets in flour, dip in beaten eggs, then press into the breadcrumb mixture.
3. Heat olive oil in a skillet over medium heat. Cook cutlets for 3–4 minutes per side until golden and crispy.
4. Drain on paper towels before serving.

Nutritional information: 360 calories, 28 g protein, 12 g carbohydrates, 20 g fat, 1 g fiber, 80 mg cholesterol, 450 mg sodium, 480 mg potassium.

Mediterranean Grilled Lamb Kebabs with Tzatziki Sauce

Yield: 4 servings | Prep time: 20 minutes | Cook time: 15 minutes

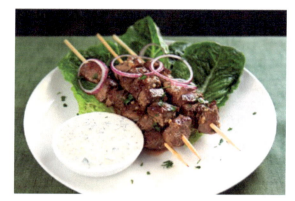

Ingredients:
For the kebabs:
- 600 g lamb leg or shoulder, cubed
- 30 ml olive oil
- 10 ml lemon juice
- 10 g garlic, minced
- 5 g paprika
- 5 g ground cumin
- 5 g dried oregano
- 5 g salt
- 2 g black pepper

For the Tzatziki sauce:
- 200 g Greek yogurt
- 100 g cucumber, grated and drained
- 10 ml lemon juice
- 10 g garlic, minced
- 10 g fresh dill, chopped
- 2 g salt

Instructions:
1. Combine lamb, olive oil, lemon juice, garlic, paprika, cumin, oregano, salt, and pepper in a bowl. Marinate for at least 1 hour.
2. Thread lamb onto skewers. Preheat the grill to medium-high heat.
3. Grill kebabs for 10–12 minutes, turning occasionally, until cooked to desired doneness.
4. Mix yogurt, cucumber, lemon juice, garlic, dill, and salt to make the Tzatziki. Serve with the kebabs.

Nutritional information: 380 calories, 32 g protein, 6 g carbohydrates, 24 g fat, 1 g fiber, 90 mg cholesterol, 500 mg sodium, 560 mg potassium.

Slow-roasted lamb Shanks in Red Wine Sauce

Yield: 4 servings | Prep time: 15 minutes | Cook time: 3 hours

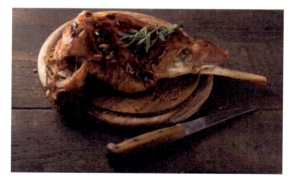

Ingredients:
- 4 lamb shanks (approximately 1.5 kg)
- 30 ml olive oil
- 1 onion, diced
- 2 carrots, diced
- 2 celery stalks, diced
- 2 cloves garlic, minced
- 300 ml red wine
- 500 ml beef stock
- 30 g tomato paste
- 2 sprigs fresh rosemary
- 2 bay leaves
- 5 g salt
- 3 g black pepper

Instructions:
1. Preheat the oven to 160°C.
2. Heat olive oil in a large ovenproof pot. Sear lamb shanks on all sides, then set aside.
3. Add onion, carrots, celery, and garlic to the pot; sauté for 5 minutes. Stir in red wine, stock, tomato paste, rosemary, bay leaves, salt, and pepper.
4. Return lamb shanks to the pot. Cover and roast in the oven for 2.5–3 hours until tender. Serve with sauce.

Nutritional information: 450 calories, 36 g protein, 10 g carbohydrates, 28 g fat, 2 g fiber, 110 mg cholesterol, 600 mg sodium, 650 mg potassium.

Spiced Lamb Kofta with Mint Yogurt Dip

Yield: 4 servings | Prep time: 15 minutes | Cook time: 15 minutes

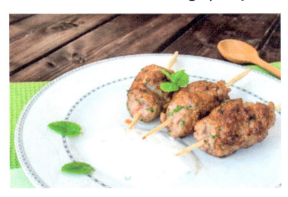

Ingredients:
For the kofta:
- 500 g ground lamb
- 10 g garlic, minced
- 5 g ground cumin
- 5 g ground coriander
- 2 g ground cinnamon
- 5 g paprika
- 5 g salt
- 2 g black pepper
- 10 g fresh parsley, chopped

For the mint yogurt dip:
- 200 g Greek yogurt
- 10 g fresh mint, chopped
- 10 ml lemon juice
- 2 g salt

Instructions:
1. Combine lamb, garlic, cumin, coriander, cinnamon, paprika, salt, pepper, and parsley in a bowl. Shape into oval patties or onto skewers.
2. Preheat a grill or skillet to medium heat. Cook kofta for 10–12 minutes, turning occasionally, until cooked.
3. Mix yogurt, mint, lemon juice, and salt to prepare the dip. Serve with the kofta.

Nutritional information: 320 calories, 28 g protein, 6 g carbohydrates, 20 g fat, 1 g fiber, 85 mg cholesterol, 520 mg sodium, 540 mg potassium.

Classic Shepherd's Pie with Ground Lamb

Yield: 6 servings | Prep time: 20 minutes | Cook time: 40 minutes

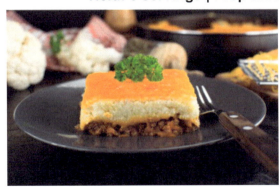

Ingredients:
- 500 g ground lamb
- 1 onion, diced
- 2 carrots, diced
- 2 cloves garlic, minced
- 200 ml beef stock
- 200 g canned diced tomatoes
- 15 ml Worcestershire sauce
- 5 g salt
- 2 g black pepper
- 500 g potatoes, peeled and cubed
- 50 g butter
- 100 ml milk

Instructions:
1. Preheat the oven to 200°C.
2. In a skillet, cook lamb until browned. Add onion, carrots, and garlic; sauté for 5 minutes.
3. Stir in stock, tomatoes, Worcestershire sauce, salt, and pepper. Simmer for 15 minutes.
4. Boil potatoes until tender. Mash with butter and milk.
5. Spread the lamb mixture in a baking dish. Top with mashed potatoes. Bake for 20 minutes until golden.

Nutritional information: 390 calories, 25 g protein, 30 g carbohydrates, 18 g fat, 3 g fiber, 85 mg cholesterol, 580 mg sodium, 620 mg potassium.

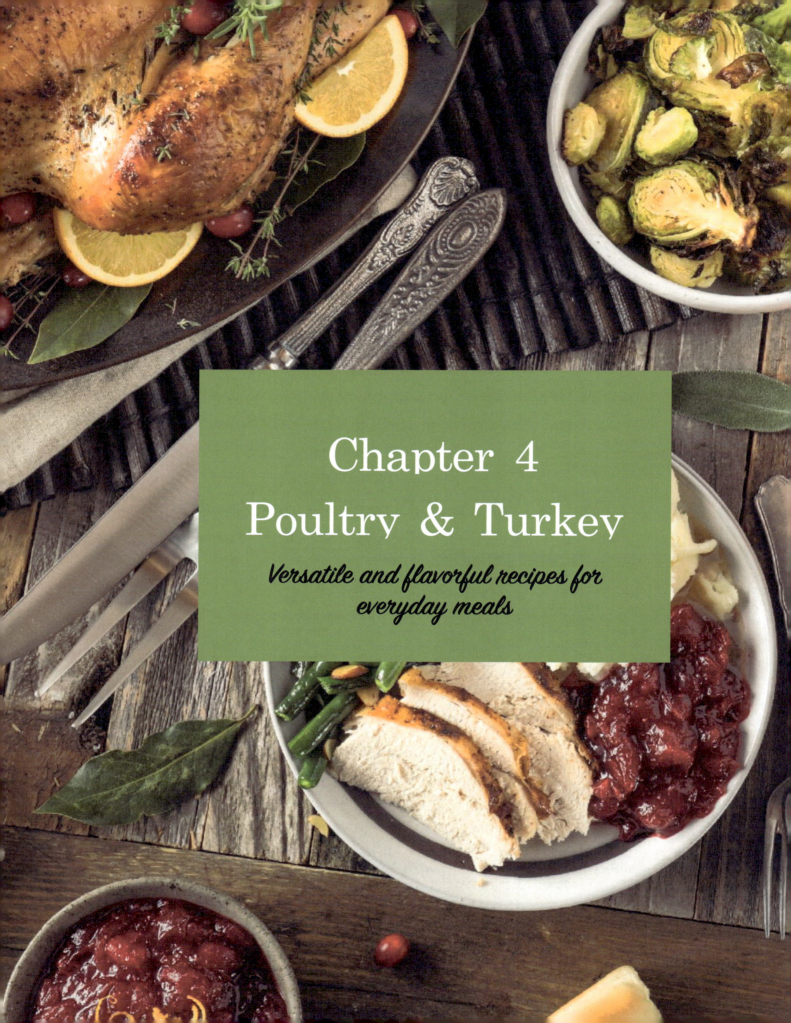

Chapter 4
Poultry & Turkey

Versatile and flavorful recipes for everyday meals

Lemon Herb Roasted Chicken Breasts

Yield: 4 servings | Prep time: 10 minutes | Cook time: 25 minutes

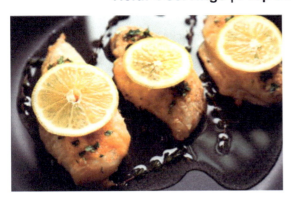

Ingredients:
- 4 boneless, skinless chicken breasts (about 150 g each)
- 30 ml olive oil
- 2 cloves garlic, minced
- Juice and zest of 1 lemon
- 10 g fresh parsley, chopped
- 5 g fresh thyme leaves
- 5 g fresh rosemary, chopped
- 1 g salt
- 0.5 g black pepper
- Optional: Lemon slices for garnish

Instructions:
1. Preheat your oven to 200°C and line a baking dish with parchment paper.
2. Mix olive oil, minced garlic, lemon juice, zest, parsley, thyme, rosemary, salt, and pepper in a small bowl.
3. Place the chicken breasts in the baking dish and rub the herb mixture all over them, ensuring an even coating.
4. Arrange lemon slices on top of the chicken if desired.
5. Bake in the preheated oven for 25 minutes or until the internal temperature of the chicken reaches 75°C.
6. Remove from the oven, rest for 5 minutes, and serve warm.

Nutritional Information:
245 calories, 30 g protein, 2 g carbohydrates, 12 g fat, 0.5 g fiber, 85 mg cholesterol, 360 mg sodium, 340 mg potassium.

Garlic Honey Glazed Chicken Thighs

Yield: 4 servings | Prep time: 10 minutes | Cook time: 30 minutes

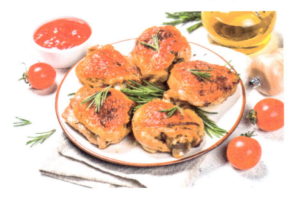

Ingredients:
- 4 chicken thighs, bone-in, skin-on (about 200 g each)
- 30 ml olive oil
- 3 cloves garlic, minced
- 30 ml honey
- 15 ml soy sauce (low sodium)
- 5 g fresh parsley, chopped (optional)

Instructions:
1. Preheat your oven to 180°C.
2. Heat olive oil in a large oven-safe skillet over medium heat. Add chicken thighs, skin-side down, and sear for 3-4 minutes until golden.
3. Flip the chicken thighs and cook for another 3 minutes.
4. In a small bowl, mix garlic, honey, and soy sauce. Pour the glaze over the chicken in the skillet.
5. Transfer the skillet to the oven and bake for 20 minutes, basting the chicken with the glaze halfway through cooking.
6. Remove from the oven, garnish with parsley if desired, and serve warm.

Nutritional Information:
320 calories, 28 g protein, 8 g carbohydrates, 18 g fat, 0.3 g fiber, 95 mg cholesterol, 400 mg sodium, 380 mg potassium.

Spicy Grilled Chicken with Cilantro Lime Sauce

Yield: 4 servings | Prep time: 15 minutes | Cook time: 10 minutes

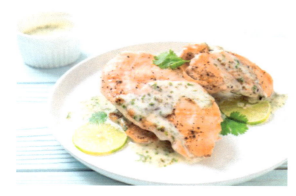

Ingredients:
- 4 boneless, skinless chicken breasts (about 150 g each)
- 15 ml olive oil
- Juice and zest of 2 limes
- 2 g chili powder
- 2 g ground cumin
- 1 g smoked paprika
- 1 g salt
- 0.5 g black pepper

Cilantro Lime Sauce:
- 50 g fresh cilantro leaves
- 30 ml olive oil
- Juice of 1 lime
- 1 clove garlic
- 15 g Greek yogurt (optional)

Instructions:
1. Mix olive oil, lime juice, zest, chili powder, cumin, paprika, salt, and pepper in a bowl. Rub the mixture onto the chicken breasts.
2. Heat a grill or grill pan over medium-high heat. Cook the chicken for 5 minutes on each side or until the internal temperature reaches 75°C.
3. For the sauce, blend cilantro, olive oil, lime juice, garlic, and Greek yogurt until smooth.
4. Serve the chicken drizzled with the cilantro lime sauce.

Nutritional Information:

260 calories, 32 g protein, 3 g carbohydrates, 12 g fat, 0.5 g fiber, 85 mg cholesterol, 350 mg sodium, 420 mg potassium.

Herbed Turkey Meatballs in Tomato Basil Sauce

Yield: 4 servings | Prep time: 20 minutes | Cook time: 30 minutes

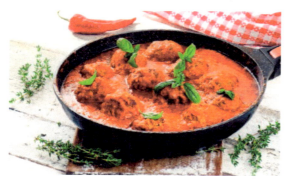

Ingredients:
- 500 g ground turkey
- 50 g breadcrumbs
- 1 egg
- 10 g fresh parsley, chopped
- 5 g dried oregano
- 1 g salt
- 0.5 g black pepper
- 15 ml olive oil
- 400 g canned crushed tomatoes
- 2 cloves garlic, minced
- 5 g fresh basil, chopped

Instructions:
1. Combine turkey, breadcrumbs, egg, parsley, oregano, salt, and pepper in a bowl. Form into 16 small meatballs.
2. Heat olive oil in a skillet over medium heat. Sear the meatballs for 5 minutes, turning occasionally, until browned.
3. Remove the meatballs and set aside. Add garlic to the skillet and sauté for 1 minute.
4. Pour in crushed tomatoes, stir in basil, and simmer. Add the meatballs back to the skillet.
5. Cover and cook for 20 minutes on low heat. Serve with your choice of side.

Nutritional Information:

290 calories, 28 g protein, 10 g carbohydrates, 12 g fat, 2 g fiber, 85 mg cholesterol, 480 mg sodium, 430 mg potassium.

Classic Chicken and Vegetable Stir-Fry

Yield: 4 servings | Prep time: 15 minutes | Cook time: 15 minutes

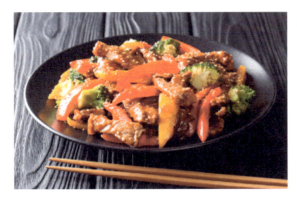

Ingredients:
- 400 g boneless, skinless chicken breast cut into thin strips
- 30 ml sesame oil
- 2 cloves garlic, minced
- 10 g fresh ginger, grated
- 1 red bell pepper, sliced
- 1 yellow bell pepper, sliced
- 1 carrot, julienned
- 100 g broccoli florets
- 50 g snap peas
- 30 ml low-sodium soy sauce
- 15 ml rice vinegar
- 5 g cornstarch mixed with 30 ml water
- 1 g salt
- 0.5 g black pepper
- Optional: Sesame seeds for garnish

Instructions:
1. Heat sesame oil in a large wok or skillet over medium-high heat.
2. Add chicken strips and cook for 4-5 minutes until browned. Remove from the wok and set aside.
3. Add garlic and ginger to the wok, sautéing for 1 minute until fragrant.
4. Add all vegetables and stir-fry for 5-7 minutes until tender-crisp.
5. Return the chicken to the wok, add soy sauce, rice vinegar, and the cornstarch slurry. Stir well to coat.
6. Cook for 2-3 minutes until the sauce thickens.
7. Serve hot, garnished with sesame seeds if desired.

Nutritional Information:
280 calories, 28 g protein, 12 g carbohydrates, 10 g fat, 3 g fiber, 85 mg cholesterol, 400 mg sodium, 420 mg potassium.

Citrus-Marinated Turkey Cutlets with Roasted Vegetables

Yield: 4 servings | Prep time: 20 minutes | Cook time: 25 minutes

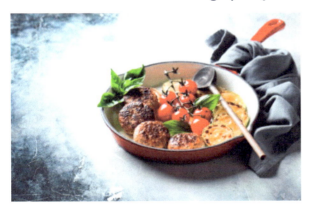

Ingredients:
- 4 turkey cutlets (about 150 g each)
- Juice and zest of 1 orange
- Juice and zest of 1 lemon
- 30 ml olive oil
- 2 cloves garlic, minced
- 1 g dried thyme
- 1 g salt
- 0.5 g black pepper
- 400 g mixed vegetables (e.g., zucchini, bell peppers, and carrots), diced

Instructions:
1. Mix orange juice, lemon juice, olive oil, garlic, thyme, salt, and pepper in a bowl. Marinate the turkey cutlets in the mixture for at least 15 minutes.
2. Preheat your oven to 200°C and line a baking sheet with parchment paper.
3. Place the marinated turkey cutlets and mixed vegetables on the sheet. Drizzle with marinade.
4. Roast for 25 minutes or until the turkey's internal temperature reaches 75°C.
5. Serve with a fresh salad or whole grains.

Nutritional Information:
250 calories, 30 g protein, 8 g carbohydrates, 10 g fat, 2 g fiber, 65 mg cholesterol, 280 mg sodium, 410 mg potassium.

Creamy Mushroom and Spinach Stuffed Chicken

Yield: 4 servings | Prep time: 15 minutes | Cook time: 30 minutes

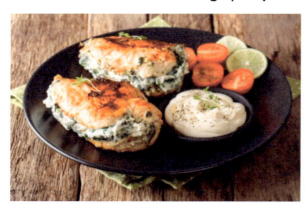

Ingredients:
- 4 boneless, skinless chicken breasts (about 150 g each)
- 30 ml olive oil
- 150 g mushrooms, finely chopped
- 100 g fresh spinach
- 30 g cream cheese
- 30 g grated Parmesan cheese
- 1 clove garlic, minced
- 1 g salt
- 0.5 g black pepper
- Optional: Fresh parsley for garnish

Instructions:
1. Preheat your oven to 190°C and lightly grease a baking dish.
2. Butterfly the chicken breasts by slicing them horizontally but not all the way through.
3. Heat 15 ml olive oil in a skillet over medium heat. Sauté mushrooms and garlic for 3-4 minutes. Add spinach and cook until wilted. Remove from heat and mix in cream cheese and Parmesan.
4. Stuff each chicken breast with the spinach-mushroom mixture and secure it with toothpicks.
5. Heat the remaining olive oil in the skillet and sear the chicken for 2-3 minutes on each side.
6. Transfer to the baking dish and bake for 20 minutes or until the internal temperature reaches 75°C.
7. Garnish with parsley and serve.

Nutritional Information:
320 calories, 35 g protein, 4 g carbohydrates, 16 g fat, 1.5 g fiber, 95 mg cholesterol, 320 mg sodium, 400 mg potassium.

Maple-glazed turkey Tenderloins with Garlic Mashed Potatoes

Yield: 4 servings | Prep time: 20 minutes | Cook time: 30 minutes

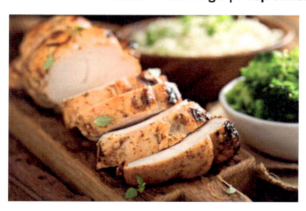

Ingredients:
- 500 g turkey tenderloins
- 30 ml maple syrup
- 15 ml Dijon mustard
- 1 clove garlic, minced
- 15 ml olive oil
- 1 g salt
- 0.5 g black pepper

Garlic Mashed Potatoes:
- 600 g potatoes, peeled and diced
- 30 ml milk (or unsweetened plant-based milk)
- 15 g butter (or vegan butter)
- 1 clove garlic, minced
- 1 g salt
- 0.5 g black pepper

Instructions:
1. Preheat your oven to 200°C and line a baking dish with parchment paper.
2. Whisk maple syrup, Dijon mustard, minced garlic, olive oil, salt, and pepper in a small bowl.
3. Place turkey tenderloins in the baking dish and brush with the maple glaze. Bake for 25-30 minutes, basting halfway through, until the internal temperature reaches 75°C.
4. While the turkey is baking, boil the potatoes in salted water for 15-20 minutes until tender. Drain and mash with milk, butter, garlic, salt, and pepper.
5. Serve the glazed turkey with garlic mashed potatoes.

Nutritional Information:
390 calories, 32 g protein, 25 g carbohydrates, 12 g fat, 3 g fiber, 85 mg cholesterol, 400 mg sodium, 450 mg potassium.

Savory Turkey Chili with Black Beans and Corn

Yield: 4 servings | Prep time: 10 minutes | Cook time: 40 minutes

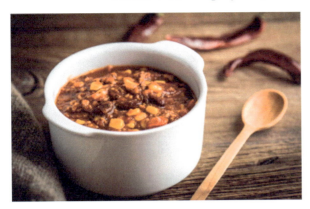

Ingredients:

- 500 g ground turkey
- 30 ml olive oil
- 1 medium onion, diced
- 2 cloves garlic, minced
- 400 g canned diced tomatoes
- 400 g canned black beans, rinsed and drained
- 200 g sweet corn kernels (fresh or canned, drained)
- 250 ml chicken broth (low sodium)
- 5 g chili powder
- 2 g ground cumin
- 1 g smoked paprika
- 0.5 g cayenne pepper (optional)
- 1 g salt
- 0.5 g black pepper
- Optional: Fresh cilantro and lime wedges for garnish

Instructions:

1. Heat olive oil in a large pot over medium heat. Add diced onion and sauté for 3-4 minutes until softened. Add garlic and cook for 1 minute.
2. Add ground turkey and cook for 5-7 minutes, breaking it up with a spoon, until browned.
3. Stir in chili powder, cumin, paprika, cayenne, salt, and black pepper. Cook for 1 minute until fragrant.
4. Add diced tomatoes, black beans, corn, and chicken broth. Stir well and bring to a boil.
5. Reduce the heat to low, cover, and simmer for 30 minutes, stirring occasionally.
6. Serve warm with fresh cilantro and lime wedges if desired.

Nutritional Information:

330 calories, 30 g protein, 20 g carbohydrates, 12 g fat, 7 g fiber, 85 mg cholesterol, 480 mg sodium, 510 mg potassium.

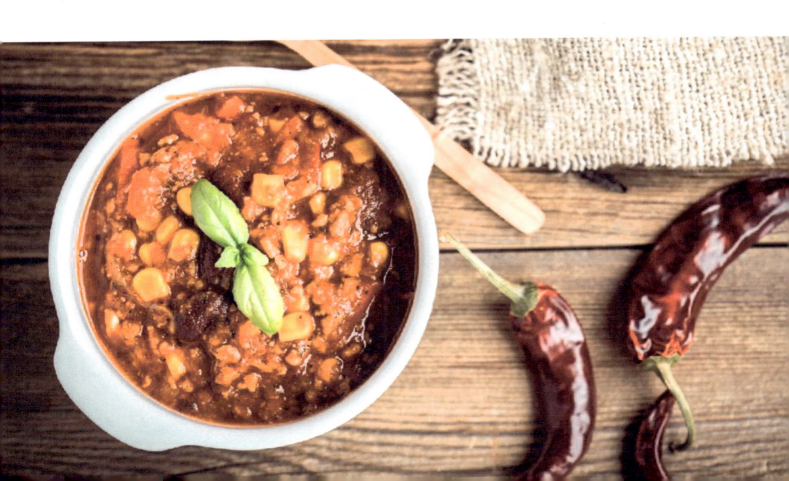

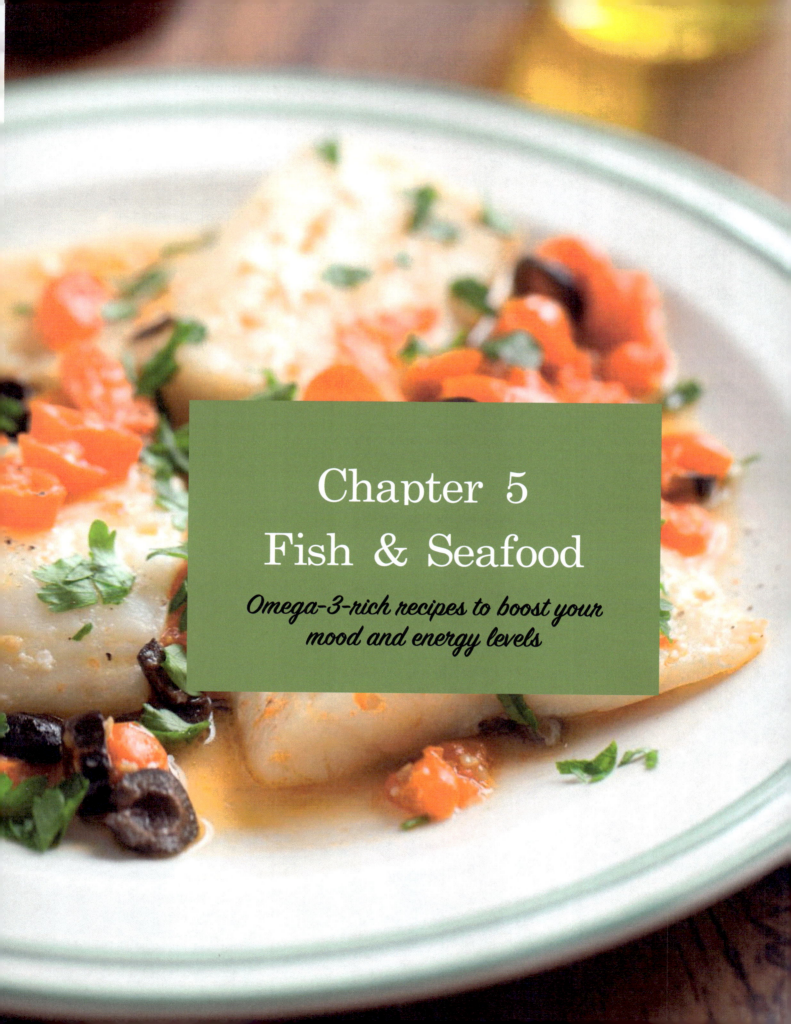

Chapter 5
Fish & Seafood

Omega-3-rich recipes to boost your mood and energy levels

Lemon Herb Salmon with Quinoa Salad

Yield: 4 servings | Prep time: 15 minutes | Cook time: 25 minutes

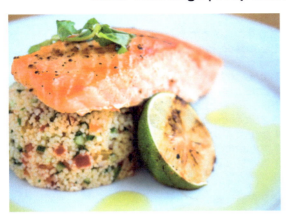

Ingredients:
- 4 salmon fillets (150 g each)
- 200 g quinoa
- 500 ml water
- 1 cucumber, diced (200 g)
- 150 g cherry tomatoes, halved
- 1 small red onion, finely chopped (80 g)
- 2 tbsp olive oil (30 ml)
- 1 lemon, juiced and zested (60 ml juice)
- 2 tbsp fresh parsley, chopped (8 g)
- 1 tsp dried oregano (2 g)
- 1 tsp salt (6 g)
- ½ tsp black pepper (2 g)

Instructions:
1. Preheat oven to 200°C. Line a baking sheet with parchment paper.
2. Place salmon fillets on the sheet and season with salt, pepper, oregano, and half the lemon juice. Bake for 15-20 minutes or until cooked through.
3. While the salmon cooks, rinse the quinoa under cold water. Combine quinoa and water in a saucepan. Bring to a boil, reduce heat, cover, and simmer for 15 minutes or until tender.
4. Combine cucumber, cherry tomatoes, red onion, parsley, olive oil, remaining lemon juice, and zest in a large bowl. Add cooked quinoa and mix well.
5. Serve salmon over quinoa salad and garnish with additional parsley if desired.

Nutritional Information: 380 calories, 36 g protein, 25 g carbohydrates, 15 g fat, 3 g fiber, 70 mg cholesterol, 480 mg sodium, 650 mg potassium.

Garlic Butter Shrimp with Zucchini Noodles

Yield: 4 servings | Prep time: 10 minutes | Cook time: 15 minutes

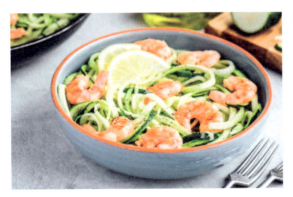

Ingredients:
- 500 g shrimp, peeled and deveined
- 3 medium zucchinis (600 g), spiralized
- 3 garlic cloves, minced (10 g)
- 2 tbsp butter (30 g)
- 2 tbsp olive oil (30 ml)
- 1 lemon, juiced (60 ml)
- 1 tsp chili flakes (2 g)
- ½ tsp salt (3 g)
- ½ tsp black pepper (2 g)

Instructions:
1. Heat olive oil and butter in a large skillet over medium heat. Add garlic and sauté until fragrant, about 1 minute.
2. Add shrimp, chili flakes, salt, and pepper. Cook for 3-5 minutes, stirring occasionally, until shrimp turn pink and are fully cooked. Remove shrimp and set aside.
3. Add zucchini noodles to the skillet and toss in the garlic butter for 2-3 minutes until slightly softened.
4. Return shrimp to the skillet, add lemon juice, and toss to combine.
5. Serve immediately, garnished with additional chili flakes if desired.

Nutritional Information: 290 calories, 28 g protein, 10 g carbohydrates, 18 g fat, 2 g fiber, 195 mg cholesterol, 520 mg sodium, 600 mg potassium.

Spicy Tuna Poke Bowl with Avocado

Yield: 2 servings | Prep time: 20 minutes | Cook time: 0 minutes

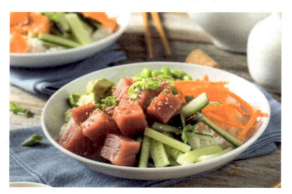

Ingredients:
- 200 g sushi-grade tuna, diced
- 1 avocado, diced (150 g)
- 150 g cooked brown rice
- 1 tbsp soy sauce (15 ml)
- 1 tbsp sesame oil (15 ml)
- 1 tsp sriracha (5 ml)
- 1 tsp sesame seeds (3 g)
- 1 green onion, sliced (10 g)
- 1 cucumber, thinly sliced (150 g)
- 1 carrot, shredded (100 g)

Instructions:
1. Combine diced tuna, soy sauce, sesame oil, sriracha, and sesame seeds in a medium bowl. Mix well and let marinate for 10 minutes.
2. Divide the cooked rice between two bowls. Top with marinated tuna, avocado, cucumber, and carrot.
3. Garnish with sliced green onion and additional sesame seeds if desired.

Nutritional Information: 410 calories, 30 g protein, 35 g carbohydrates, 16 g fat, 5 g fiber, 60 mg cholesterol, 520 mg sodium, 750 mg potassium.

Crispy Baked Cod with Sweet Potato Wedges

Yield: 4 servings | Prep time: 15 minutes | Cook time: 30 minutes

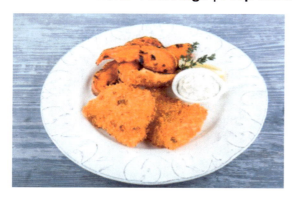

Ingredients:
- 4 cod fillets (150 g each)
- 2 large sweet potatoes, cut into wedges (500 g)
- 2 tbsp olive oil (30 ml)
- 50 g breadcrumbs
- 2 tbsp grated Parmesan cheese (10 g)
- 1 tsp paprika (2 g)
- 1 tsp garlic powder (2 g)
- ½ tsp salt (3 g)
- ½ tsp black pepper (2 g)

Instructions:
1. Preheat oven to 200°C. Line a baking sheet with parchment paper.
2. Toss sweet potato wedges with 1 tbsp olive oil, paprika, and half the salt and pepper. Spread on the baking sheet and bake for 15 minutes.
3. Meanwhile, mix breadcrumbs, Parmesan, garlic powder, and remaining salt and pepper in a small bowl. Brush cod fillets with remaining olive oil and coat with breadcrumb mixture.
4. Push sweet potatoes to one side of the baking sheet and place cod fillets on the other side. Bake for 15 minutes or until the fish is cooked through and flaky.
5. Serve cod with sweet potato wedges and garnish with fresh parsley if desired.

Nutritional Information: 320 calories, 28 g protein, 30 g carbohydrates, 10 g fat, 4 g fiber, 70 mg cholesterol, 480 mg sodium, 750 mg potassium.

Mediterranean Grilled Octopus with Fresh Herbs

Yield: 4 servings | Prep time: 20 minutes | Cook time: 45 minutes

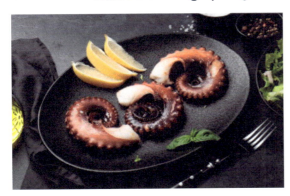

Ingredients:
- 1 kg octopus, cleaned
- 2 tbsp olive oil (30 ml)
- 2 tbsp red wine vinegar (30 ml)
- 1 lemon, juiced and zested (60 ml juice)
- 2 garlic cloves, minced (10 g)
- 2 tbsp fresh parsley, chopped (8 g)
- 1 tsp dried oregano (2 g)
- ½ tsp salt (3 g)
- ½ tsp black pepper (2 g)

Instructions:
1. Bring a large pot of salted water to a boil. Add the octopus and cook for 30 minutes until tender. Remove, drain, and cool slightly.
2. Preheat a grill or grill pan to medium-high heat.
3. Mix olive oil, vinegar, lemon juice, garlic, parsley, oregano, salt, and pepper in a small bowl.
4. Brush the octopus with half the marinade and grill for 8-10 minutes, turning occasionally, until lightly charred.
5. Slice the octopus and drizzle with the remaining marinade before serving.

Nutritional Information: 220 calories, 35 g protein, 3 g carbohydrates, 6 g fat, 0 g fiber, 160 mg cholesterol, 420 mg sodium, 750 mg potassium.

Garlic Butter Shrimp with Spinach and Cherry Tomatoes

Yield: 4 servings | Prep time: 10 minutes | Cook time: 15 minutes

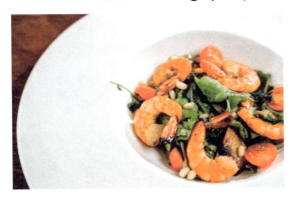

Ingredients:
- 500 g shrimp, peeled and deveined
- 2 cups fresh spinach (150 g)
- 150 g cherry tomatoes, halved
- 3 garlic cloves, minced (10 g)
- 2 tbsp butter (30 g)
- 2 tbsp olive oil (30 ml)
- ½ tsp salt (3 g)
- ½ tsp black pepper (2 g)

Instructions:
1. Heat olive oil and butter in a large skillet over medium heat. Add garlic and sauté for 1 minute.
2. Add shrimp, salt, and pepper. Cook for 3-5 minutes, stirring occasionally, until shrimp turn pink and are fully cooked.
3. Add spinach and cherry tomatoes to the skillet and toss for 2-3 minutes until spinach is wilted.
4. Serve immediately as a light main course or side dish.

Nutritional Information: 290 calories, 25 g protein, 8 g carbohydrates, 18 g fat, 2 g fiber, 195 mg cholesterol, 460 mg sodium, 650 mg potassium.

Classic Mussels in White Wine Sauce

Yield: 4 servings | Prep time: 10 minutes | Cook time: 15 minutes

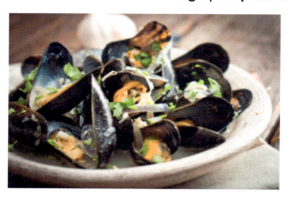

Ingredients:
- 1 kg fresh mussels, cleaned
- 2 tbsp olive oil (30 ml)
- 1 small onion, finely chopped (80 g)
- 3 garlic cloves, minced (10 g)
- 200 ml dry white wine
- 150 ml heavy cream
- 2 tbsp fresh parsley, chopped (8 g)
- ½ tsp salt (3 g)
- ½ tsp black pepper (2 g)

Instructions:
1. Heat olive oil in a large pot over medium heat. Add onion and garlic, sautéing until softened, about 3 minutes.
2. Pour in white wine and bring to a simmer. Add mussels, cover, and cook for 5-7 minutes until mussels open. Discard any that do not open.
3. Stir in cream, parsley, salt, and pepper. Simmer for 2 minutes.
4. Serve mussels with crusty bread and the white wine sauce.

Nutritional Information: 350 calories, 24 g protein, 8 g carbohydrates, 20 g fat, 0 g fiber, 60 mg cholesterol, 720 mg sodium, 550 mg potassium.

Lobster Tails with Lemon Herb Butter

Yield: 4 servings | Prep time: 10 minutes | Cook time: 20 minutes

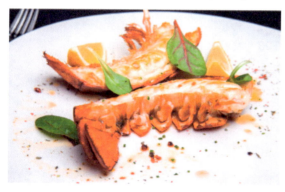

Ingredients:
- 4 lobster tails (150 g each)
- 100 g unsalted butter, melted
- 1 lemon, juiced and zested (60 ml juice)
- 2 garlic cloves, minced (10 g)
- 2 tbsp fresh parsley, chopped (8 g)
- 1 tsp paprika (2 g)
- ½ tsp salt (3 g)
- ½ tsp black pepper (2 g)

Instructions:
1. Preheat oven to 200°C. Using kitchen scissors, cut through the top shell of each lobster tail and gently pull the meat out to rest on top of the shell.
2. Mix melted butter, lemon juice, zest, garlic, parsley, paprika, salt, and pepper in a small bowl.
3. Brush the lobster meat with half the butter mixture. Place it on a baking sheet and bake for 12-15 minutes or until the meat is opaque and cooked through.
4. Serve with the remaining butter mixture for dipping.

Nutritional Information: 350 calories, 27 g protein, 3 g carbohydrates, 26 g fat, 0 g fiber, 140 mg cholesterol, 480 mg sodium, 420 mg potassium.

Scallop and Mango Ceviche

Yield: 4 servings | Prep time: 15 minutes | Cook time: 0 minutes

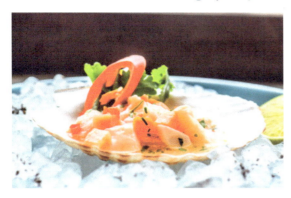

Ingredients:
- 500 g fresh scallops, diced
- 1 mango, diced (200 g)
- 1 red bell pepper, diced (150 g)
- 1 small red onion, finely chopped (80 g)
- 2 limes, juiced (120 ml)
- 1 tbsp olive oil (15 ml)
- 1 tbsp fresh cilantro, chopped (5 g)
- ½ tsp salt (3 g)
- ½ tsp black pepper (2 g)

Instructions:
1. Combine diced scallops, mango, red bell pepper, and red onion in a large bowl.
2. Pour lime juice and olive oil over the mixture. Add cilantro, salt, and pepper, and toss gently.
3. Cover and refrigerate for 30 minutes to allow the flavors to meld. Serve chilled.

Nutritional Information: 220 calories, 22 g protein, 18 g carbohydrates, 6 g fat, 2 g fiber, 30 mg cholesterol, 320 mg sodium, 550 mg potassium.

Shrimp and Avocado Salad with Lime Dressing

Yield: 4 servings | Prep time: 15 minutes | Cook time: 5 minutes

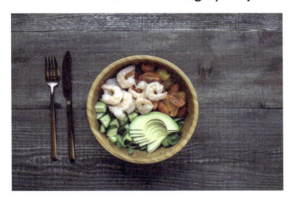

Ingredients:
- 500 g shrimp, peeled and deveined
- 2 avocados, diced (300 g)
- 150 g cherry tomatoes, halved
- 1 cucumber, diced (200 g)
- 2 tbsp olive oil (30 ml)
- 2 limes, juiced (120 ml)
- 1 tsp honey (5 ml)
- 1 garlic clove, minced (5 g)
- ½ tsp salt (3 g)
- ½ tsp black pepper (2 g)
-

Instructions:
1. Heat 1 tbsp olive oil in a skillet over medium heat. Add shrimp, salt, pepper, and sauté for 3-5 minutes until fully cooked. Let cool slightly.
2. Combine avocado, cherry tomatoes, cucumber, and cooked shrimp in a large bowl.
3. Whisk lime juice, remaining olive oil, honey, and garlic in a small bowl. Pour over the salad and toss gently to coat.
4. Serve immediately, garnished with additional lime wedges if desired.

Nutritional Information: 320 calories, 25 g protein, 12 g carbohydrates, 20 g fat, 5 g fiber, 190 mg cholesterol, 360 mg sodium, 700 mg potassium.

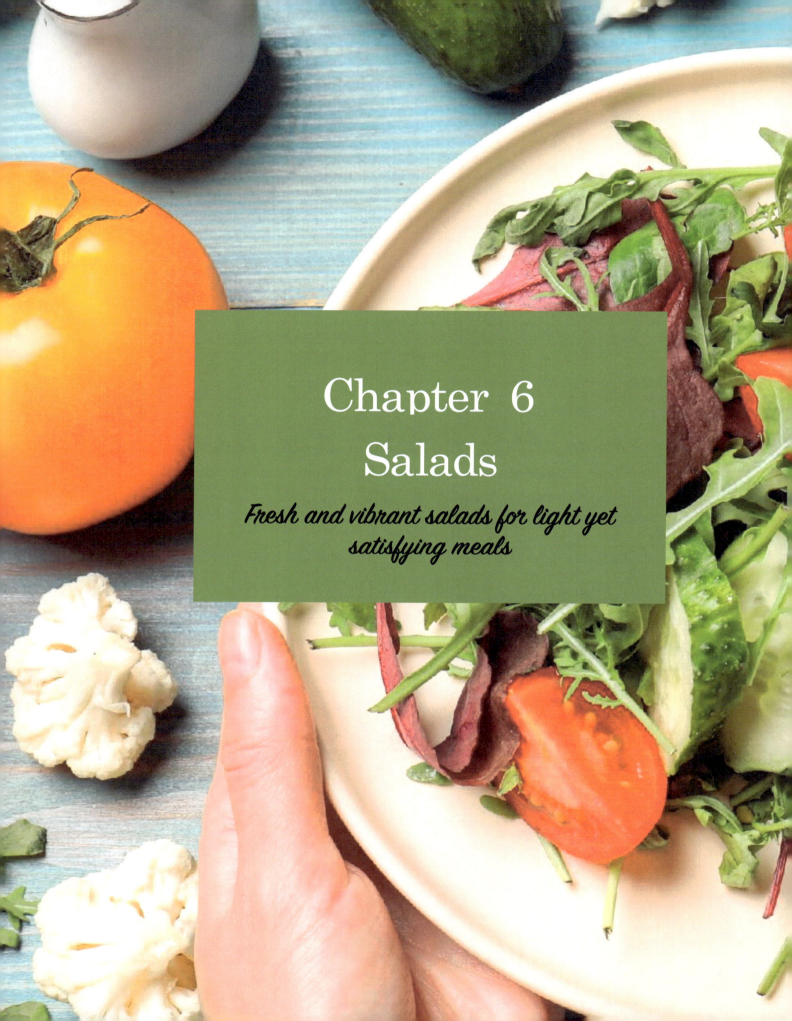

Chapter 6
Salads

Fresh and vibrant salads for light yet satisfying meals

Mediterranean Chickpea Salad with Lemon-Tahini Dressing

Yield: 4 servings | Prep time: 15 minutes | Cook time: 0 minutes

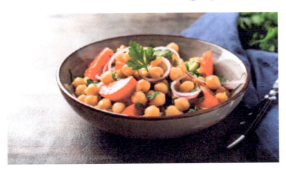

Ingredients:
- 240 g cooked chickpeas (drained and rinsed)
- 150 g cherry tomatoes, halved
- 100 g cucumber, diced
- 80 g red bell pepper, diced
- 50 g red onion, finely sliced
- 50 g Kalamata olives, pitted and sliced
- 30 g fresh parsley, chopped

For the dressing:
- 50 g tahini
- 30 ml fresh lemon juice
- 10 ml olive oil
- 5 ml water (to thin, if necessary)
- 1 garlic clove, minced
- 1 g ground cumin
- Salt and pepper to taste

Instructions:
1. Combine chickpeas, cherry tomatoes, cucumber, red bell pepper, red onion, olives, and parsley in a large bowl.
2. Whisk together tahini, lemon juice, olive oil, garlic, cumin, salt, and pepper in a small bowl. Adjust consistency with water if needed.
3. Pour dressing over the salad and toss until evenly coated. Serve immediately.

Nutritional information: 234 calories, 7 g protein, 20 g carbohydrates, 12 g fat, 6 g fiber, 0 mg cholesterol, 370 mg sodium, 260 mg potassium.

Crispy Kale Caesar Salad with a Twist of Garlic

Yield: 4 servings | Prep time: 20 minutes | Cook time: 10 minutes

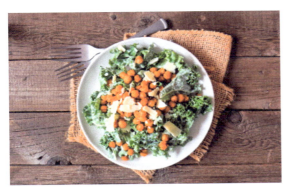

Ingredients:
- 150 g kale, stems removed and leaves torn
- 50 g roasted chickpeas (for crunch, replacing croutons)
- 20 g Parmesan cheese, grated

For the dressing:
- 50 g plain Greek yogurt
- 20 g Dijon mustard
- 10 ml lemon juice
- 10 ml olive oil
- 1 garlic clove, minced
- Salt and pepper to taste

Instructions:
1. Preheat oven to 180°C. Spread kale on a baking tray and bake for 10 minutes until crispy.
2. Combine crispy kale, roasted chickpeas, and Parmesan cheese in a large bowl.
3. Whisk together yogurt, mustard, lemon juice, olive oil, garlic, salt, and pepper in a small bowl.
4. Drizzle dressing over the salad, toss gently, and serve.

Nutritional information: 190 calories, 8 g protein, 14 g carbohydrates, 10 g fat, 5 g fiber, 4 mg cholesterol, 280 mg sodium, 220 mg potassium.

Zesty Quinoa and Avocado Salad with Lime Vinaigrette

Yield: 4 servings | Prep time: 15 minutes | Cook time: 15 minutes

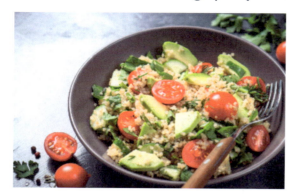

Ingredients:
- 200 g cooked quinoa
- 150 g avocado, diced
- 100 g cherry tomatoes, halved
- 50 g red onion, finely diced
- 30 g fresh cilantro, chopped

For the dressing:
- 30 ml lime juice
- 10 ml olive oil
- 1 garlic clove, minced
- Salt and pepper to taste

Instructions:
1. Cook quinoa according to package instructions. Let cool.
2. Combine quinoa, avocado, cherry tomatoes, red onion, and cilantro in a large bowl.
3. Whisk together lime juice, olive oil, garlic, salt, and pepper in a small bowl.
4. Pour dressing over the salad and toss gently to combine.

Nutritional information: 215 calories, 6 g protein, 26 g carbohydrates, 10 g fat, 5 g fiber, 0 mg cholesterol, 200 mg sodium, 310 mg potassium.

Rainbow Veggie Salad with Creamy Yogurt Dill Dressing

Yield: 4 servings | Prep time: 20 minutes | Cook time: 0 minutes

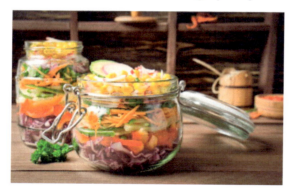

Ingredients:
- 100 g red cabbage, shredded
- 100 g carrots, julienned
- 100 g cucumber, sliced
- 80 g red bell pepper, diced
- 50 g sweet corn (canned, drained)
- 30 g fresh dill, chopped

For the dressing:
- 100 g plain Greek yogurt
- 10 ml lemon juice
- 5 ml olive oil
- 1 garlic clove, minced
- Salt and pepper to taste

Instructions:
1. Combine red cabbage, carrots, cucumber, red bell pepper, sweet corn, and dill in a large bowl.
2. Whisk together yogurt, lemon juice, olive oil, garlic, salt, and pepper in a small bowl.
3. Pour the dressing over the vegetables and toss until well coated. Serve immediately.

Nutritional information: 145 calories, 5 g protein, 20 g carbohydrates, 6 g fat, 4 g fiber, 2 mg cholesterol, 190 mg sodium, 270 mg potassium.

Watermelon and Feta Salad with Mint and Balsamic Drizzle

Yield: 4 servings | Prep time: 15 minutes | Cook time: 0 minutes

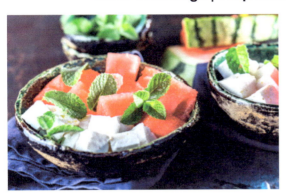

Ingredients:
- 400 g watermelon, cubed
- 100 g feta cheese, crumbled
- 30 g fresh mint leaves, chopped
- 10 ml balsamic glaze

Instructions:
1. Combine watermelon, feta cheese, and mint leaves in a large bowl.
2. Drizzle balsamic glaze over the salad. Toss gently to combine and serve chilled.

Nutritional information: 172 calories, 6 g protein, 18 g carbohydrates, 8 g fat, 1 g fiber, 22 mg cholesterol, 220 mg sodium, 210 mg potassium.

Lentil and Arugula Salad with Honey-Mustard Dressing

Yield: 4 servings | Prep time: 15 minutes | Cook time: 10 minutes

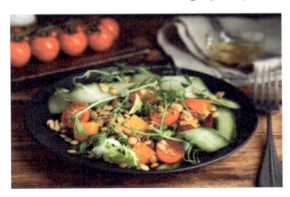

Ingredients:
- 240 g cooked lentils (drained and rinsed)
- 100 g arugula
- 100 g cherry tomatoes, halved
- 50 g cucumber, diced
- 30 g red onion, thinly sliced

For the dressing:
- 10 ml Dijon mustard
- 10 ml honey
- 10 ml apple cider vinegar
- 10 ml olive oil
- Salt and pepper to taste

Instructions:
1. Combine lentils, arugula, cherry tomatoes, cucumber, and red onion in a large bowl.
2. Whisk together Dijon mustard, honey, apple cider vinegar, olive oil, salt, and pepper in a small bowl.
3. Pour the dressing over the salad and toss gently. Serve immediately.

Nutritional information: 215 calories, 10 g protein, 28 g carbohydrates, 7 g fat, 6 g fiber, 0 mg cholesterol, 210 mg sodium, 290 mg potassium.

Asian-Inspired Cabbage Slaw with Sesame-Ginger Dressing

Yield: 4 servings | Prep time: 15 minutes | Cook time: 0 minutes

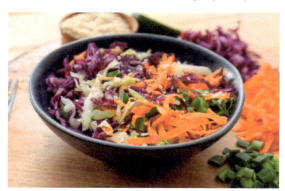

Ingredients:
- 200 g green cabbage, shredded
- 100 g red cabbage, shredded
- 50 g carrots, julienned
- 30 g green onions, sliced
- 10 g sesame seeds

For the dressing:
- 10 ml sesame oil
- 20 ml rice vinegar
- 10 ml soy sauce
- 5 ml honey
- 5 ml grated fresh ginger

Instructions:
1. Combine green cabbage, red cabbage, carrots, and green onions in a large bowl.
2. Whisk together sesame oil, rice vinegar, soy sauce, honey, and ginger in a small bowl.
3. Pour the dressing over the slaw and toss to combine. Garnish with sesame seeds. Serve immediately.

Nutritional information: 152 calories, 3 g protein, 15 g carbohydrates, 9 g fat, 4 g fiber, 0 mg cholesterol, 250 mg sodium, 210 mg potassium.

Hearty Spinach and Strawberry Salad with Toasted Almonds

Yield: 4 servings | Prep time: 15 minutes | Cook time: 5 minutes

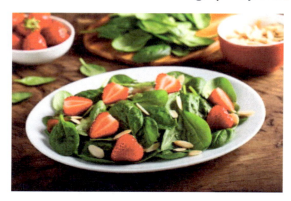

Ingredients:
For the Salad:
- 150 g fresh spinach leaves, washed and dried
- 200 g strawberries, hulled and sliced
- 50 g crumbled goat cheese (optional)
- 50 g sliced almonds
- 50 g red onion, thinly sliced

For the Poppy Seed Dressing:
- 60 ml olive oil
- 30 ml apple cider vinegar
- 15 g honey
- 5 g Dijon mustard
- 5 g poppy seeds
- Salt, to taste
- Freshly ground black pepper, to taste

Instructions:
1. Heat a small skillet over medium heat. Add sliced almonds and toast for 2–3 minutes, stirring frequently, until golden and fragrant. Remove from heat and set aside.
2. Whisk together olive oil, apple cider vinegar, honey, Dijon mustard, poppy seeds, salt, and pepper in a small bowl until well combined. Adjust seasoning to taste.
3. In a large salad bowl, combine spinach leaves, sliced strawberries, red onion, and goat cheese (if using).
4. Sprinkle the toasted almonds over the salad. Drizzle the poppy seed dressing evenly over the top.
5. Gently toss the salad to combine all the ingredients. Serve immediately as a side or light main course.

Nutritional Information
Per serving: 240 calories, 5 g protein, 16 g carbohydrates, 18 g fat, 4 g fiber, 5 mg cholesterol, 90 mg sodium, 420 mg potassium.

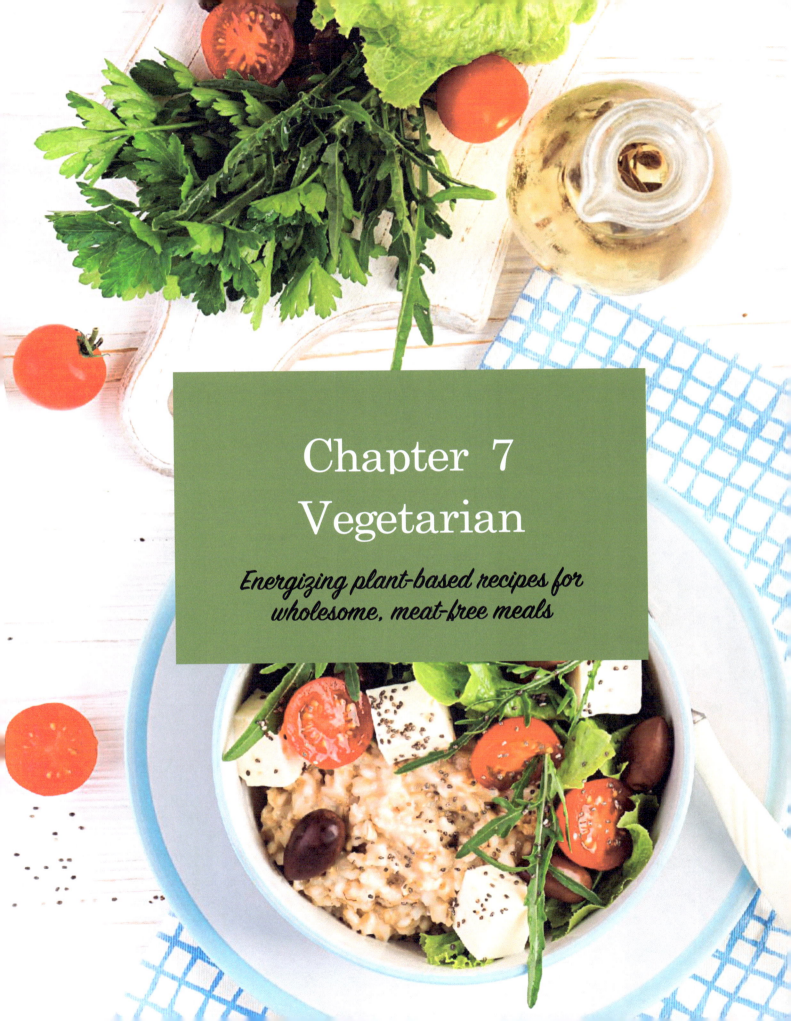

Chapter 7
Vegetarian

Energizing plant-based recipes for wholesome, meat-free meals

Grilled Eggplant with Garlic Yogurt Sauce

Yield: 4 servings | Prep time: 15 minutes | Cook time: 20 minutes

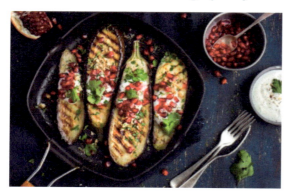

Ingredients:
- 2 medium eggplants (approx. 600 g)
- 30 ml olive oil
- 200 g plain Greek yogurt
- 1 clove garlic, minced
- 10 ml lemon juice
- 5 g fresh parsley, chopped
- Salt and pepper to taste

Instructions:
1. Preheat the grill to medium heat.
2. Slice eggplants into 1 cm thick rounds. Brush both sides with olive oil and season with salt and pepper.
3. Grill eggplant slices for 8–10 minutes per side or until tender and slightly charred.
4. Mix Greek yogurt, garlic, lemon juice, and a pinch of salt in a small bowl.
5. Arrange grilled eggplant on a platter and drizzle with garlic yogurt sauce. Garnish with parsley and serve.

Nutritional Information

123 calories, 3.7 g protein, 11.8 g carbohydrates, 7.8 g fat, 4.3 g fiber, 0 mg cholesterol, 88 mg sodium, 312 mg potassium.

Crispy Zucchini Fritters with Dill Dip

Yield: 4 servings | Prep time: 20 minutes | Cook time: 15 minutes

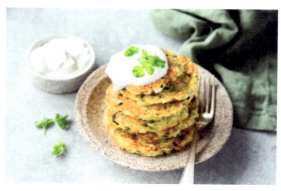

Ingredients:
- 500 g zucchini, grated
- 5 g salt
- 60 g all-purpose flour
- 2 large eggs
- 10 g fresh dill, chopped
- 30 ml olive oil (for frying)
- 100 g plain Greek yogurt
- 5 g garlic, minced
- 5 g fresh dill (for dip)

Instructions:
1. Grate zucchini, sprinkle with salt, and let sit for 10 minutes. Squeeze out excess liquid.
2. Combine zucchini, flour, eggs, and dill to form a batter.
3. Heat olive oil in a skillet over medium heat. Drop spoonfuls of batter into the pan, flattening slightly. Cook for 3–4 minutes per side until golden.
4. Mix the yogurt, garlic, and dill to prepare the dip.
5. Serve fritters warm with dill dip.

Nutritional Information

142 calories, 6.1 g protein, 10.2 g carbohydrates, 9.1 g fat, 1.5 g fiber, 55 mg cholesterol, 222 mg sodium, 298 mg potassium.

Baked Spinach and Feta Stuffed Portobello Mushrooms

Yield: 4 servings | Prep time: 15 minutes | Cook time: 20 minutes

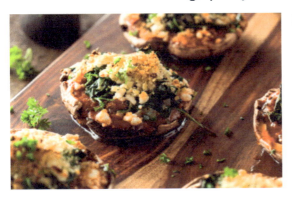

Ingredients:
- 4 large portobello mushrooms (approx. 400 g)
- 200 g fresh spinach
- 100 g feta cheese, crumbled
- 30 g breadcrumbs
- 15 ml olive oil
- 5 g garlic, minced
- Salt and pepper to taste

Instructions:
1. Preheat oven to 200°C. Remove stems from mushrooms and hollow out caps slightly.
2. Heat olive oil in a pan, sauté garlic and spinach until wilted. Season with salt and pepper.
3. Mix sautéed spinach with feta and breadcrumbs.
4. Stuff mushroom caps with the mixture and place on a baking tray. Bake for 15–20 minutes.
5. Serve warm as a side or main dish.

Nutritional Information

163 calories, 8.9 g protein, 7.4 g carbohydrates, 11.2 g fat, 2.1 g fiber, 18 mg cholesterol, 275 mg sodium, 490 mg potassium.

Creamy Tomato and Basil Risotto

Yield: 4 servings | Prep time: 10 minutes | Cook time: 25 minutes

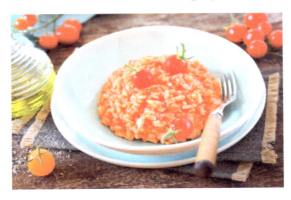

Ingredients:
- 200 g Arborio rice
- 30 ml olive oil
- 1 small onion, finely chopped (100 g)
- 2 cloves garlic, minced
- 120 ml dry white wine
- 500 ml vegetable stock, warmed
- 200 g canned crushed tomatoes
- 30 g Parmesan cheese, grated
- 10 g fresh basil leaves, chopped
- Salt and pepper to taste

Instructions:
1. Heat olive oil in a large pan over medium heat. Sauté onion and garlic until softened.
2. Stir in Arborio rice and cook for 2 minutes until coated in oil.
3. Add white wine and cook until absorbed. Gradually add warm vegetable stock, stirring constantly, until rice is creamy and tender (about 20 minutes).
4. Stir in crushed tomatoes, Parmesan, and basil—season with salt and pepper.
5. Serve immediately, garnished with extra basil.

Nutritional Information

287 calories, 7.8 g protein, 47.2 g carbohydrates, 7.5 g fat, 2.6 g fiber, 9 mg cholesterol, 305 mg sodium, and 310 mg potassium.

Broccoli and Cashew Stir-Fry with Ginger Soy Sauce

Yield: 4 servings | Prep time: 15 minutes | Cook time: 15 minutes

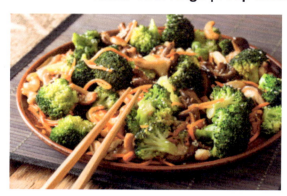

Ingredients:
- 300 g broccoli florets
- 100 g carrots, julienned
- 75 g unsalted cashews
- 15 ml sesame oil
- 2 cloves garlic, minced
- 5 g fresh ginger, grated
- 30 ml soy sauce
- 15 ml rice vinegar
- 5 g cornflour mixed with 15 ml water
- 15 g green onions, chopped

Instructions:
1. Heat sesame oil in a wok or large pan over medium-high heat. Stir-fry garlic and ginger for 1 minute.
2. Add broccoli and carrots. Stir-fry for 5 minutes until tender-crisp.
3. Stir in soy sauce, rice vinegar, and cashews. Add cornflour mixture and cook until sauce thickens.
4. Garnish with green onions and serve over steamed rice or noodles.

Nutritional Information

202 calories, 6.5 g protein, 17.6 g carbohydrates, 11.3 g fat, 3.8 g fiber, 0 mg cholesterol, 474 mg sodium, 290 mg potassium.

Sweet Potato and Kale Hash with a Poached Egg

Yield: 2 servings | Prep time: 15 minutes | Cook time: 20 minutes

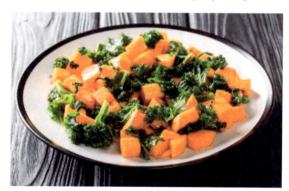

Ingredients:
- 300 g sweet potatoes, peeled and diced
- 100 g kale, chopped
- 15 ml olive oil
- 2 cloves garlic, minced
- 2 large eggs
- Salt and pepper to taste
- 5 g fresh parsley, chopped

Instructions:
1. Heat olive oil in a skillet over medium heat. Add sweet potatoes and cook for 10 minutes until golden and tender.
2. Add garlic and kale, cooking for 5 minutes until wilted. Season with salt and pepper.
3. In a separate pot, poach eggs in simmering water for 3–4 minutes.
4. Serve sweet potato hash topped with a poached egg and garnish with parsley.

Nutritional Information

245 calories, 9.4 g protein, 28.2 g carbohydrates, 10.3 g fat, 4.8 g fiber, 186 mg cholesterol, 126 mg sodium, 400 mg potassium.

Vegan Pad Thai with Peanut Sauce

Yield: 4 servings | Prep time: 15 minutes | Cook time: 15 minutes

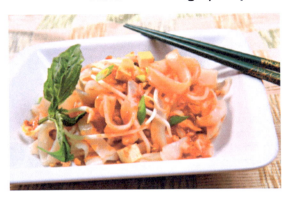

Ingredients:
- 200 g rice noodles
- 150 g firm tofu, cubed
- 15 ml sesame oil
- 100 g bean sprouts
- 50 g carrots, julienned
- 30 g green onions, chopped
- 30 g roasted peanuts, chopped
- 60 ml peanut butter
- 30 ml soy sauce
- 15 ml lime juice
- 10 g brown sugar
- 5 g chili flakes (optional)

Instructions:
1. Cook rice noodles according to package instructions and set aside.
2. Heat sesame oil in a skillet over medium heat. Sauté tofu until golden.
3. Mix peanut butter, soy sauce, lime juice, sugar, and chili flakes in a bowl. Add a bit of warm water to thin the sauce.
4. Add noodles, tofu, bean sprouts, and carrots to the skillet. Toss with peanut sauce until evenly coated.
5. Garnish with green onions and peanuts. Serve warm.

Nutritional Information
322 calories, 12.3 g protein, 43.5 g carbohydrates, 12.1 g fat, 3.5 g fiber, 0 mg cholesterol, 496 mg sodium, 412 mg potassium.

Roasted Beet and Arugula Salad with Citrus Dressing

Yield: 4 servings | Prep time: 15 minutes | Cook time: 40 minutes

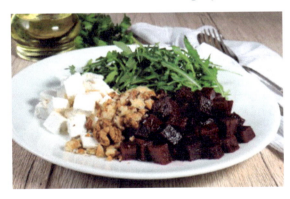

Ingredients:
- 500 g beets, peeled and quartered
- 15 ml olive oil
- 100 g arugula
- 50 g walnuts, toasted
- 50 g goat cheese, crumbled
- 30 ml orange juice
- 15 ml lemon juice
- 10 ml honey
- 10 ml olive oil (for dressing)
- Salt and pepper to taste

Instructions:
1. Preheat the oven to 200°C. Toss the beets with olive oil, salt, and pepper, then roast on a baking tray for 35–40 minutes or until tender.
2. Whisk orange juice, lemon juice, honey, and olive oil in a small bowl for the dressing.
3. Arrange arugula on a serving platter. Top with roasted beets, walnuts, and goat cheese.
4. Drizzle with citrus dressing and serve immediately.

Nutritional Information
198 calories, 6.8 g protein, 17.5 g carbohydrates, 11.3 g fat, 4.1 g fiber, 6 mg cholesterol, 103 mg sodium, and 472 mg potassium.

Mediterranean Orzo Salad with Olives and Feta

Yield: 4 servings | Prep time: 15 minutes | Cook time: 10 minutes

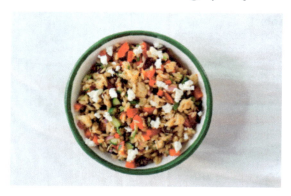

Ingredients:
- 200 g orzo pasta
- 150 g cherry tomatoes, halved
- 50 g black olives, sliced
- 50 g cucumber, diced
- 50 g feta cheese, crumbled
- 15 g fresh parsley, chopped
- 30 ml olive oil
- 15 ml red wine vinegar
- 5 g dried oregano
- Salt and pepper to taste

Instructions:
1. Cook orzo according to package instructions. Drain and let cool.
2. Combine cooked orzo, cherry tomatoes, olives, cucumber, feta, and parsley in a large bowl.
3. Whisk olive oil, vinegar, oregano, salt, and pepper in a small bowl. Pour over the salad and toss to combine.
4. Chill for 15 minutes before serving.

Nutritional Information

275 calories, 7.1 g protein, 32.4 g carbohydrates, 11.5 g fat, 2.1 g fiber, 9 mg cholesterol, 342 mg sodium, 224 mg potassium.

Homemade Veggie Burgers with Avocado Spread

Yield: 4 servings | Prep time: 20 minutes | Cook time: 15 minutes

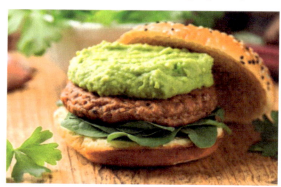

Ingredients:
- 400 g cooked black beans, mashed
- 100 g breadcrumbs
- 50 g carrots, grated
- 50 g onions, finely chopped
- 15 ml olive oil
- 1 clove garlic, minced
- 1 tsp cumin powder
- 1 avocado
- 10 ml lemon juice
- 4 whole-grain burger buns

Instructions:
1. Mix mashed black beans, breadcrumbs, carrots, onions, garlic, and cumin until well combined. Shape into four patties.
2. Heat olive oil in a skillet over medium heat. Cook patties for 5–7 minutes per side until golden brown.
3. Mash avocado with lemon juice and a pinch of salt in a small bowl.
4. Assemble burgers with buns, veggie patties, and avocado spread. Serve warm.

Nutritional Information

315 calories, 9.2 g protein, 38.3 g carbohydrates, 11.2 g fat, 8.3 g fiber, 0 mg cholesterol, 245 mg sodium, 516 mg potassium.

Cauliflower Steaks with Chimichurri Sauce

Yield: 4 servings | Prep time: 15 minutes | Cook time: 20 minutes

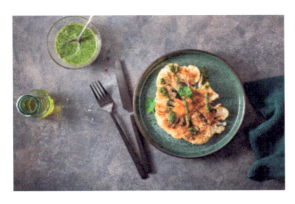

Ingredients:

- 1 large cauliflower (approx. 700 g)
- 30 ml olive oil
- Salt and pepper to taste
- 15 g fresh parsley, chopped
- 10 g fresh cilantro, chopped
- 10 ml red wine vinegar
- 10 ml lemon juice
- 1 clove garlic, minced
- 60 ml olive oil (for sauce)

Instructions:

1. Preheat oven to 200°C. Cut cauliflower into 2 cm thick steaks. Brush both sides with olive oil and season with salt and pepper.
2. Place on a baking sheet and roast for 20 minutes, flipping halfway through, until golden and tender.
3. Mix parsley, cilantro, garlic, vinegar, lemon juice, and olive oil in a bowl to make the chimichurri sauce.
4. Drizzle sauce over roasted cauliflower steaks and serve warm.

Nutritional Information

186 calories, 3.2 g protein, 9.3 g carbohydrates, 15.1 g fat, 4.2 g fiber, 0 mg cholesterol, 82 mg sodium, 489 mg potassium.

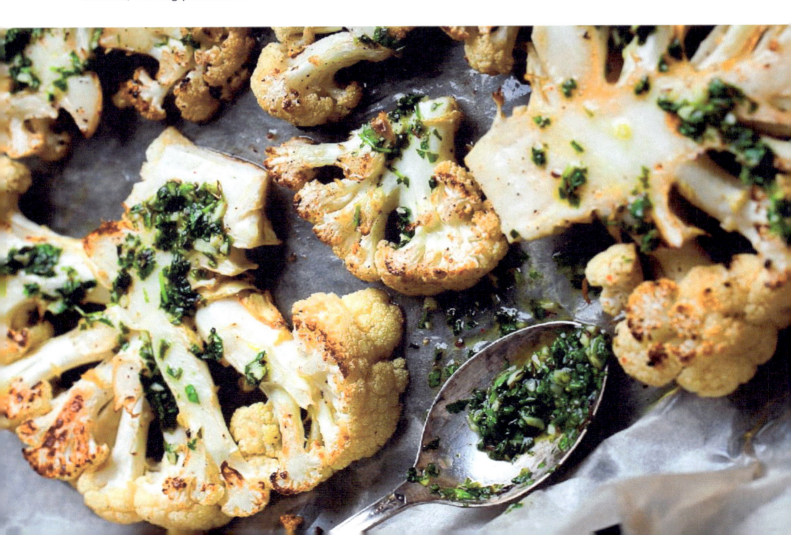

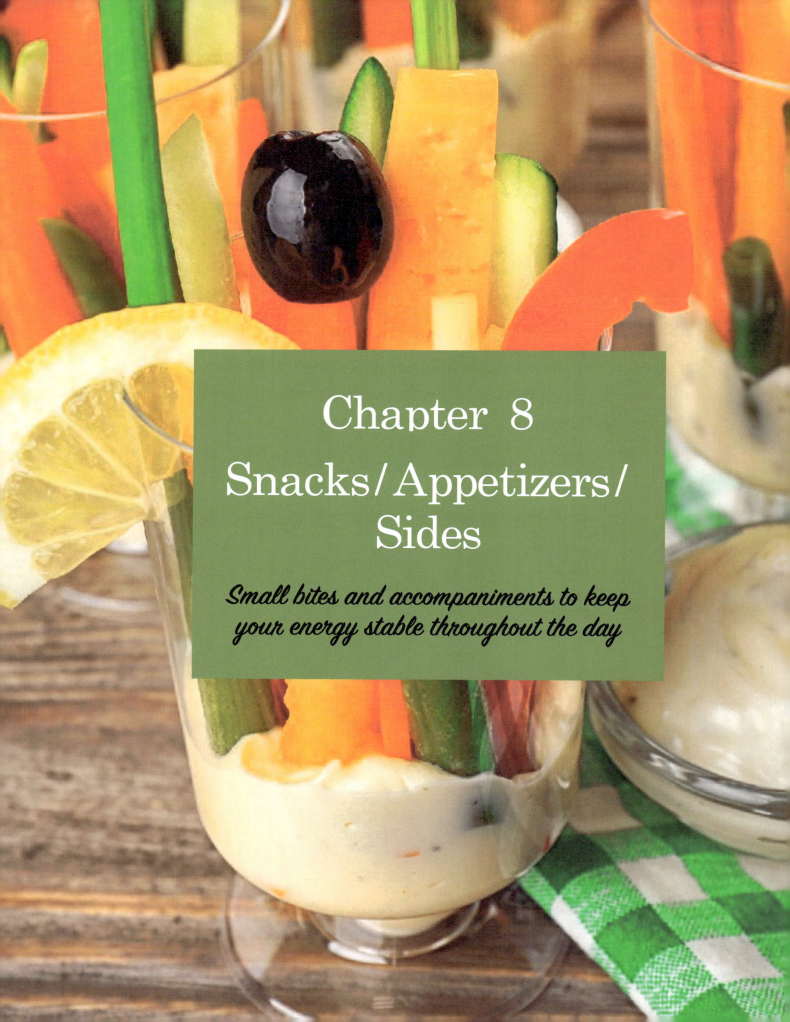

Chapter 8
Snacks/Appetizers/Sides

*Small bites and accompaniments to keep
your energy stable throughout the day*

Crunchy Chickpea Snack Bites

Yield: 4 servings | Prep time: 10 minutes | Cook time: 30 minutes

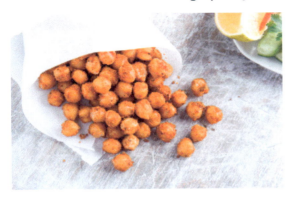

Ingredients:
- 400 g canned chickpeas, drained and rinsed
- 15 ml olive oil
- 5 g smoked paprika
- 3 g ground cumin
- 2 g garlic powder
- 1 g salt
- 1 g black pepper

Instructions:
1. Preheat the oven to 200°C.
2. Pat the chickpeas dry with a paper towel.
3. Mix chickpeas, olive oil, smoked paprika, cumin, garlic powder, salt, and pepper in a mixing bowl. Toss to coat evenly.
4. Spread chickpeas on a baking sheet in a single layer.
5. Roast for 30 minutes, stirring halfway through, until crispy.
6. Let cool before serving.

Nutritional information: 135 calories, 6 g protein, 18 g carbohydrates, 4 g fat, 5 g fiber, 0 mg cholesterol, 240 mg sodium, 230 mg potassium.

Savory Sweet Potato Wedges with Spicy Yogurt Dip

Yield: 4 servings | Prep time: 10 minutes | Cook time: 25 minutes

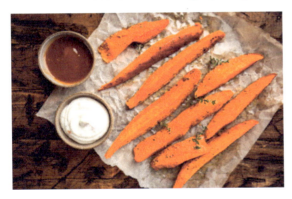

Ingredients:
For Sweet Potato Wedges:
- 600 g sweet potatoes, cut into wedges
- 15 ml olive oil
- 5 g smoked paprika
- 2 g garlic powder
- 2 g salt
- 1 g black pepper

For Spicy Yogurt Dip:
- 120 g plain Greek yogurt
- 5 ml hot sauce
- 5 ml lemon juice
- 1 g salt

Instructions:
1. Preheat oven to 220°C.
2. Toss sweet potato wedges with olive oil, smoked paprika, garlic powder, salt, and pepper. Spread evenly on a baking sheet.
3. Bake for 25 minutes, flipping halfway through.
4. Mix yogurt, hot sauce, lemon juice, and salt in a small bowl for the dip.
5. Serve wedges with the spicy yogurt dip.

Nutritional information: 175 calories, 4 g protein, 30 g carbohydrates, 4 g fat, 4 g fiber, 5 mg cholesterol, 230 mg sodium, 300 mg potassium.

Herbed Quinoa-Stuffed Bell Peppers

Yield: 4 servings | Prep time: 15 minutes | Cook time: 30 minutes

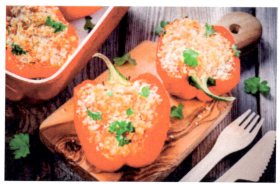

Ingredients:
- 4 bell peppers, halved and deseeded
- 150 g quinoa
- 300 ml vegetable broth
- 50 g cherry tomatoes, diced
- 30 g feta cheese, crumbled
- 15 g parsley, chopped
- 2 g dried oregano
- 2 g salt
- 1 g black pepper

Instructions:
1. Preheat oven to 190°C.
2. Cook quinoa in vegetable broth according to package instructions.
3. Mix cooked quinoa, tomatoes, feta, parsley, oregano, salt, and pepper in a bowl.
4. Stuff bell pepper halves with the quinoa mixture.
5. Place peppers on a baking sheet and bake for 30 minutes.

Nutritional information: 190 calories, 7 g protein, 30 g carbohydrates, 4 g fat, 4 g fiber, 10 mg cholesterol, 270 mg sodium, 350 mg potassium.

Zesty Avocado and Black Bean Salsa

Yield: 4 servings | Prep time: 10 minutes | Cook time: 0 minutes

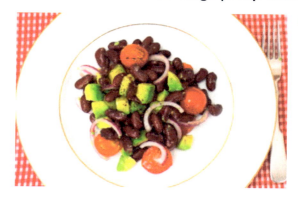

Ingredients:
- 200 g black beans, cooked and rinsed
- 1 ripe avocado, diced
- 100 g cherry tomatoes, diced
- 50 g red onion, finely chopped
- 15 ml lime juice
- 15 g fresh cilantro, chopped
- 2 g salt
- 1 g black pepper

Instructions:
1. Combine black beans, avocado, cherry tomatoes, red onion, lime juice, and cilantro in a mixing bowl.
2. Add salt and pepper, and gently toss to combine.
3. Serve immediately with tortilla chips or as a topping for grilled dishes.

Nutritional information: 160 calories, 4 g protein, 20 g carbohydrates, 7 g fat, 7 g fiber, 0 mg cholesterol, 240 mg sodium, 350 mg potassium.

Mediterranean-Style Hummus Platter with Veggie Sticks

Yield: 4 servings | Prep time: 15 minutes | Cook time: 0 minutes

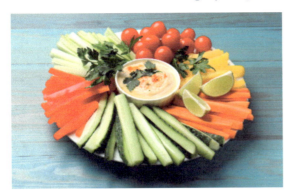

Ingredients:
For the Hummus:
- 400 g canned chickpeas, drained and rinsed
- 30 ml olive oil
- 30 ml tahini
- 15 ml lemon juice
- 1 clove garlic, minced
- 2 g salt
- 30 ml water (as needed for consistency)

For the Veggie Sticks:
- 1 cucumber, cut into sticks
- 2 carrots, cut into sticks
- 1 red bell pepper, sliced
- 1 yellow bell pepper, sliced
- 15 cherry tomatoes
- 1 celery, cut into sticks

Instructions:
1. Blend chickpeas, olive oil, tahini, lemon juice, garlic, and salt in a food processor until smooth. Add water to achieve the desired consistency.
2. Arrange the hummus in the center of a platter and surround it with vegetable sticks.
3. Serve immediately.

Nutritional information: 220 calories, 6 g protein, 20 g carbohydrates, 10 g fat, 7 g fiber, 0 mg cholesterol, 320 mg sodium, 400 mg potassium.

Mini Cucumber and Smoked Salmon Bites

Yield: 4 servings | Prep time: 10 minutes | Cook time: 0 minutes

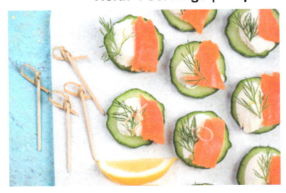

Ingredients:
- 1 cucumber, sliced into rounds
- 100 g smoked salmon, cut into small strips
- 50 g cream cheese
- 5 g fresh dill, chopped
- 5 ml lemon juice

Instructions:
1. Spread a small amount of cream cheese on each cucumber round.
2. Top with a strip of smoked salmon.
3. Garnish with dill and a squeeze of lemon juice.
4. Serve immediately as a fresh appetizer.

Nutritional information: 90 calories, 6 g protein, 2 g carbohydrates, 6 g fat, 1 g fiber, 15 mg cholesterol, 180 mg sodium, 150 mg potassium.

Oven-roasted garlic Parmesan Cauliflower

Yield: 4 servings | Prep time: 10 minutes | Cook time: 25 minutes

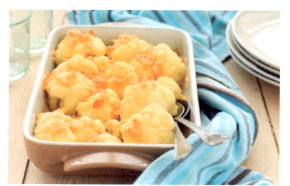

Ingredients:
- 500 g cauliflower florets
- 15 ml olive oil
- 20 g grated Parmesan cheese
- 1 clove garlic, minced
- 2 g salt
- 1 g black pepper

Instructions:
1. Preheat oven to 200°C.
2. Toss cauliflower florets with olive oil, Parmesan cheese, garlic, salt, and pepper.
3. Spread evenly on a baking sheet and roast for 25 minutes, stirring halfway through.
4. Serve warm as a flavorful side dish.

Nutritional information: 110 calories, 5 g protein, 8 g carbohydrates, 6 g fat, 3 g fiber, 5 mg cholesterol, 240 mg sodium, 300 mg potassium.

Lentil and Spinach Energy Balls

Yield: 4 servings | Prep time: 15 minutes | Cook time: 0 minutes

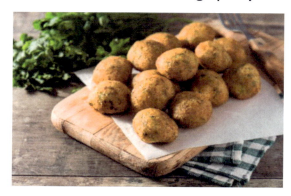

Ingredients:
- 150 g cooked lentils
- 50 g spinach, finely chopped
- 30 g rolled oats
- 10 g sunflower seeds
- 15 ml olive oil
- 2 g salt
- 1 g black pepper

Instructions:
1. Combine lentils, spinach, oats, sunflower seeds, olive oil, salt, and pepper in a food processor. Blend until the mixture holds together.
2. Roll into bite-sized balls.
3. Chill in the refrigerator for 30 minutes before serving.

Nutritional information: 120 calories, 6 g protein, 15 g carbohydrates, 3 g fat, 4 g fiber, 0 mg cholesterol, 200 mg sodium, 270 mg potassium.

Baked Zucchini Chips with Lemon-Herb Dip

Yield: 4 servings | Prep time: 10 minutes | Cook time: 25 minutes

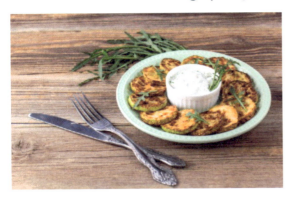

Ingredients:
For Zucchini Chips:
- 2 medium zucchinis, sliced into thin rounds
- 15 ml olive oil
- 10 g breadcrumbs
- 10 g grated Parmesan cheese
- 2 g salt
- 1 g black pepper

For Lemon-Herb Dip:
- 120 g plain Greek yogurt
- 5 ml lemon juice
- 5 g fresh parsley, chopped
- 1 g garlic powder
- 1 g salt

Instructions:
1. Preheat oven to 200°C.
2. Toss zucchini slices with olive oil, breadcrumbs, Parmesan, salt, and pepper. Spread on a baking sheet.
3. Bake for 25 minutes, flipping halfway through, until crispy.
4. Mix yogurt, lemon juice, parsley, garlic powder, and salt for the dip.
5. Serve chips warm with the dip.

Nutritional information: 150 calories, 5 g protein, 12 g carbohydrates, 7 g fat, 2 g fiber, 5 mg cholesterol, 220 mg sodium, 300 mg potassium.

Crispy Kale Chips with Nutritional Yeast

Yield: 4 servings | Prep time: 10 minutes | Cook time: 15 minutes

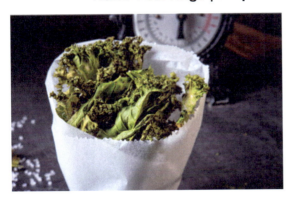

Ingredients:
- 200 g fresh kale, stems removed and torn into pieces
- 15 ml olive oil
- 15 g nutritional yeast
- 2 g salt
-

Instructions:
1. Preheat oven to 180°C.
2. Wash and thoroughly dry kale pieces.
3. Toss kale with olive oil, nutritional yeast, and salt in a mixing bowl until evenly coated.
4. Spread kale on a baking sheet in a single layer.
5. Bake for 15 minutes, flipping halfway through, until crispy.
6. Allow to cool slightly before serving.

Nutritional information: 90 calories, 4 g protein, 8 g carbohydrates, 4 g fat, 2 g fiber, 0 mg cholesterol, 150 mg sodium, 300 mg potassium.

Roasted Beet and Goat Cheese Salad Cups

Yield: 4 servings | Prep time: 15 minutes | Cook time: 40 minutes

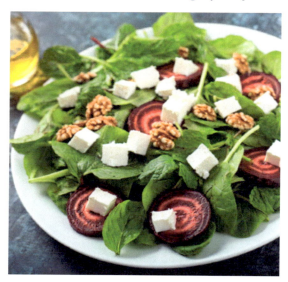

Ingredients:
- 300 g beets, peeled and diced
- 15 ml olive oil
- 2 g salt
- 50 g goat cheese, crumbled
- 50 g walnuts, chopped
- 10 g fresh mint, chopped
- 4 butter lettuce leaves (for serving)

Instructions:
1. Preheat oven to 200°C.
2. Toss beets with olive oil and salt. Roast on a baking sheet for 40 minutes, stirring halfway through, until tender.
3. Allow beets to cool slightly, then mix with goat cheese, walnuts, and mint.
4. Serve the mixture in butter lettuce leaves as cups.

Nutritional information: 190 calories, 5 g protein, 15 g carbohydrates, 12 g fat, 3 g fiber, 10 mg cholesterol, 150 mg sodium, 300 mg potassium.

Spicy Edamame Pods with Sea Salt and Lime

Yield: 4 servings | Prep time: 5 minutes | Cook time: 10 minutes

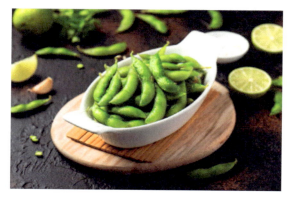

Ingredients:
- 400 g edamame pods, frozen
- 5 ml sesame oil
- 5 ml soy sauce
- 2 g chili flakes
- 2 g sea salt
- 15 ml lime juice

Instructions:
1. Boil edamame in salted water for 5 minutes. Drain and set aside.
2. Heat sesame oil in a skillet over medium heat. Add edamame, soy sauce, chili flakes, and sea salt. Stir-fry for 5 minutes.
3. Remove from heat and drizzle with lime juice before serving.

Nutritional information: 140 calories, 8 g protein, 11 g carbohydrates, 7 g fat, 5 g fiber, 0 mg cholesterol, 290 mg sodium, 300 mg potassium.

Mushroom and Herb Polenta Bites

Yield: 4 servings | Prep time: 15 minutes | Cook time: 25 minutes

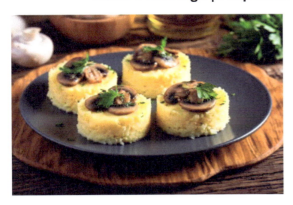

Ingredients:
- 150 g polenta
- 600 ml water
- 10 g butter
- 2 g salt
- 150 g mushrooms, diced
- 10 ml olive oil
- 5 g fresh thyme, chopped

Instructions:
1. In a saucepan, bring water to a boil and gradually add polenta while stirring. Cook for 10 minutes, then stir in butter and salt.
2. Spread polenta onto a lined baking sheet, smoothing it to about 1 cm thick. Cool and cut into small rounds.
3. In a skillet, sauté mushrooms in olive oil until golden, about 5 minutes. Add thyme and cook for two more minutes.
4. Top polenta rounds with mushrooms and serve warm.

Nutritional information: 170 calories, 4 g protein, 25 g carbohydrates, 6 g fat, 2 g fiber, 10 mg cholesterol, 150 mg sodium, 250 mg potassium.

Wholesome Trail Mix Energy Clusters

Yield: 6 servings | Prep time: 10 minutes | Cook time: 15 minutes

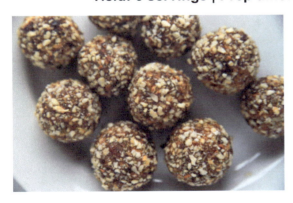

Ingredients:
- 100 g rolled oats
- 50 g almonds, chopped
- 50 g dried cranberries
- 30 g dark chocolate chips
- 60 ml honey
- 15 ml almond butter

Instructions:
1. Preheat oven to 180°C.
2. Mix oats, almonds, cranberries, and chocolate chips in a bowl.
3. In a saucepan, heat honey and almond butter over low heat until combined. Pour over dry ingredients and mix well.
4. Scoop the mixture into small clusters on a baking sheet. Bake for 15 minutes.
5. Let cool before serving or storing.

Nutritional information: 190 calories, 4 g protein, 26 g carbohydrates, 8 g fat, 3 g fiber, 0 mg cholesterol, 30 mg sodium, 150 mg potassium.

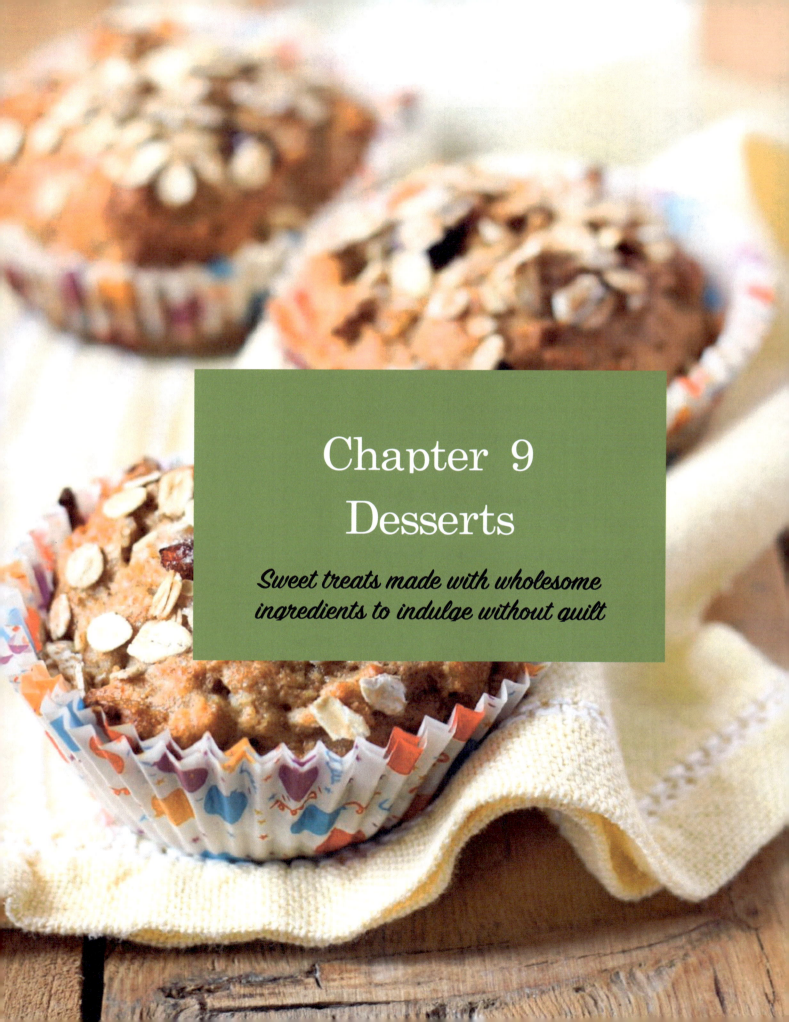

Chapter 9
Desserts

Sweet treats made with wholesome ingredients to indulge without guilt

Dark Chocolate Avocado Mousse

Yield: 4 servings | Prep time: 10 minutes | Cook time: 0 minutes

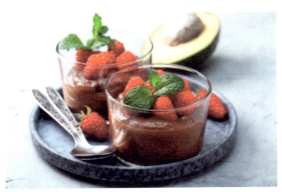

Ingredients:
- 2 ripe avocados (about 300 g), peeled and pitted
- 60 g dark chocolate (70% cocoa), melted
- 30 g cocoa powder
- 30 ml maple syrup
- 5 ml vanilla extract
- 2 g salt

Instructions:
1. Blend avocados, melted dark chocolate, cocoa powder, maple syrup, vanilla extract, and salt in a food processor until smooth.
2. Divide the mousse into serving dishes and chill for at least 30 minutes before serving.

Nutritional information: 220 calories, 3 g protein, 19 g carbohydrates, 16 g fat, 7 g fiber, 0 mg cholesterol, 50 mg sodium, 370 mg potassium.

Coconut Chia Pudding with Fresh Berries

Yield: 4 servings | Prep time: 5 minutes | Cook time: 0 minutes (plus chilling time)

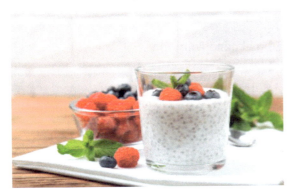

Ingredients:
- 400 ml coconut milk
- 60 g chia seeds
- 30 ml maple syrup
- 200 g mixed fresh berries (e.g., blueberries, raspberries, strawberries)

Instructions:
1. Whisk together coconut milk, chia seeds, and maple syrup in a bowl.
2. Cover and refrigerate for at least 4 hours or overnight, stirring occasionally to prevent clumping.
3. Serve topped with fresh berries.

Nutritional information: 210 calories, 4 g protein, 14 g carbohydrates, 15 g fat, 8 g fiber, 0 mg cholesterol, 20 mg sodium, 220 mg potassium.

Oatmeal Energy Cookies with Almond Butter

Yield: 6 servings | Prep time: 10 minutes | Cook time: 15 minutes

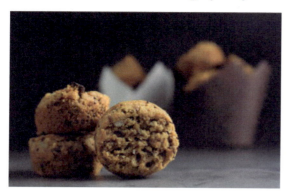

Ingredients:
- 150 g rolled oats
- 100 g almond butter
- 50 g honey
- 50 g dark chocolate chips
- 30 g chopped almonds
- 5 g cinnamon
- 1 g salt

Instructions:
1. Preheat oven to 180°C.
2. Mix oats, almond butter, honey, chocolate chips, almonds, cinnamon, and salt until well combined.
3. Scoop dough into small balls and flatten slightly on a baking sheet.
4. Bake for 15 minutes or until golden brown. Allow to cool before serving.

Nutritional information: 210 calories, 5 g protein, 22 g carbohydrates, 12 g fat, 4 g fiber, 0 mg cholesterol, 35 mg sodium, 170 mg potassium.

Lemon Blueberry Greek Yogurt Bars

Yield: 6 servings | Prep time: 15 minutes | Cook time: 30 minutes

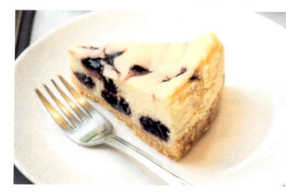

Ingredients:
For the Base:
- 150 g rolled oats
- 50 g almond flour
- 30 ml honey
- 15 ml coconut oil, melted

For the Filling:
- 300 g Greek yogurt
- 2 eggs
- 50 ml lemon juice
- 30 g honey
- 100 g fresh blueberries

Instructions:
1. Preheat oven to 175°C. Line a baking dish with parchment paper.
2. Mix oats, almond flour, honey, and coconut oil for the base. Press into the dish and bake for 10 minutes.
3. Whisk Greek yogurt, eggs, lemon juice, and honey in a bowl. Pour over the baked base and top with blueberries.
4. Bake for 20 minutes or until set. Chill before cutting into bars.

Nutritional information: 180 calories, 8 g protein, 20 g carbohydrates, 7 g fat, 2 g fiber, 30 mg cholesterol, 40 mg sodium, 130 mg potassium.

Banana Nice Cream with Peanut Swirl

Yield: 4 servings | Prep time: 5 minutes | Cook time: 0 minutes

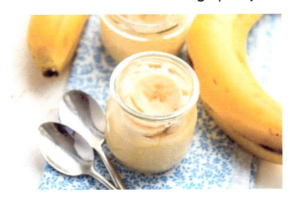

Ingredients:
- 4 ripe bananas (about 400 g), sliced and frozen
- 30 g peanut butter
- 5 ml vanilla extract

Instructions:
1. Blend frozen bananas and vanilla extract in a food processor until smooth.
2. Swirl in peanut butter with a spoon.
3. Serve immediately or freeze for a firmer texture.

Nutritional information: 150 calories, 3 g protein, 30 g carbohydrates, 4 g fat, 3 g fiber, 0 mg cholesterol, 20 mg sodium, 400 mg potassium.

Quinoa Chocolate Chip Protein Bites

Yield: 6 servings | Prep time: 10 minutes | Cook time: 15 minutes

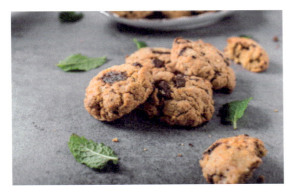

Ingredients:
- 150 g cooked quinoa
- 50 g rolled oats
- 50 g almond butter
- 30 g dark chocolate chips
- 30 ml honey
- 5 g chia seeds

Instructions:
1. Preheat oven to 180°C.
2. Mix a bowl of quinoa, oats, almond butter, chocolate chips, honey, and chia seeds.
3. Roll the mixture into bite-sized balls and place on a baking sheet.
4. Bake for 15 minutes. Cool before serving.

Nutritional information: 160 calories, 4 g protein, 20 g carbohydrates, 6 g fat, 3 g fiber, 0 mg cholesterol, 30 mg sodium, 150 mg potassium.

Apple Cinnamon Crumble with Oat Topping

Yield: 4 servings | Prep time: 10 minutes | Cook time: 25 minutes

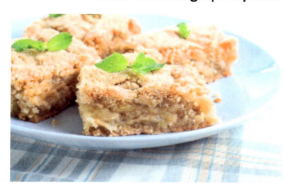

Ingredients:
For the Filling:
- 4 apples (about 400 g), peeled, cored, and sliced
- 5 g cinnamon
- 15 ml maple syrup

For the Topping:
- 100 g rolled oats
- 50 g almond flour
- 30 g coconut oil, melted
- 15 g chopped walnuts

Instructions:
1. Preheat oven to 190°C.
2. Toss apples with cinnamon and maple syrup. Spread in a baking dish.
3. Mix oats, almond flour, coconut oil, and walnuts for the topping. Sprinkle over apples.
4. Bake for 25 minutes or until golden and bubbly.

Nutritional information: 210 calories, 3 g protein, 30 g carbohydrates, 9 g fat, 4 g fiber, 0 mg cholesterol, 10 mg sodium, 180 mg potassium.

Matcha Green Tea Bliss Balls

Yield: 4 servings | Prep time: 10 minutes | Cook time: 0 minutes

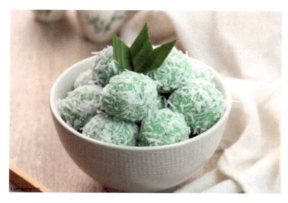

Ingredients:
- 100 g rolled oats
- 50 g almond flour
- 30 ml maple syrup
- 15 g coconut oil, melted
- 5 g matcha powder
- 20 g shredded coconut (for rolling)

Instructions:
1. Combine oats, almond flour, maple syrup, coconut oil, and matcha powder in a mixing bowl. Mix until the dough holds together.
2. Roll into bite-sized balls.
3. Coat each ball with shredded coconut.
4. Chill in the refrigerator for at least 30 minutes before serving.

Nutritional information: 120 calories, 3 g protein, 15 g carbohydrates, 6 g fat, 2 g fiber, 0 mg cholesterol, 10 mg sodium, 70 mg potassium.

Dark Chocolate Avocado Truffles

Yield: 4 servings | Prep time: 15 minutes | Cook time: 0 minutes

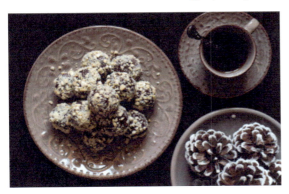

Ingredients:
- 2 ripe avocados (about 300 g), peeled and pitted
- 100 g dark chocolate (70% cocoa), melted
- 30 g cocoa powder
- 10 g powdered sugar
- 20 g shredded coconut or crushed nuts (optional for coating)

Instructions:
1. Blend avocados, melted dark chocolate, cocoa powder, and powdered sugar in a food processor until smooth.
2. Chill the mixture in the refrigerator for 30 minutes.
3. Scoop and roll the mixture into small balls.
4. Roll each ball in shredded coconut or crushed nuts.
5. Store in the fridge until ready to serve.

Nutritional information: 170 calories, 2 g protein, 14 g carbohydrates, 12 g fat, 4 g fiber, 0 mg cholesterol, 15 mg sodium, 300 mg potassium.

Peanut Butter Banana Protein Muffins

Yield: 6 servings | Prep time: 10 minutes | Cook time: 20 minutes

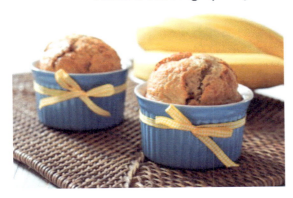

Ingredients:
- 2 ripe bananas (about 200 g), mashed
- 100 g rolled oats
- 50 g peanut butter
- 2 eggs
- 10 g chia seeds
- 5 g baking powder
- 5 g cinnamon

Instructions:
1. Preheat oven to 180°C.
2. Combine mashed bananas, oats, peanut butter, eggs, chia seeds, baking powder, and cinnamon in a mixing bowl. Mix until smooth.
3. Divide the batter into a lined muffin tin.
4. Bake for 20 minutes or until golden brown and a toothpick comes out clean.
5. Cool before serving.

Nutritional information: 190 calories, 6 g protein, 20 g carbohydrates, 8 g fat, 3 g fiber, 30 mg cholesterol, 110 mg sodium, 250 mg potassium.

Sweet Potato Brownies

Yield: 6 servings | Prep time: 10 minutes | Cook time: 25 minutes

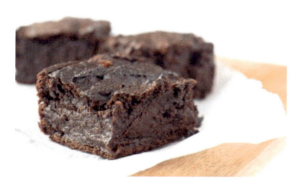

Ingredients:
- 300 g sweet potatoes, cooked and mashed
- 50 g almond flour
- 50 g cocoa powder
- 30 ml maple syrup
- 15 ml coconut oil, melted
- 2 eggs
- 5 g baking powder

Instructions:
1. Preheat oven to 180°C. Line a baking dish with parchment paper.
2. Mix mashed sweet potatoes, almond flour, cocoa powder, maple syrup, coconut oil, eggs, and baking powder until smooth.
3. Pour the mixture into the baking dish and spread evenly.
4. Bake for 25 minutes or until set. Let cool before slicing.

Nutritional information: 180 calories, 5 g protein, 22 g carbohydrates, 8 g fat, 3 g fiber, 30 mg cholesterol, 50 mg sodium, 250 mg potassium.

Chocolate Coconut Energy Bars

Yield: 6 servings | Prep time: 10 minutes | Cook time: 0 minutes

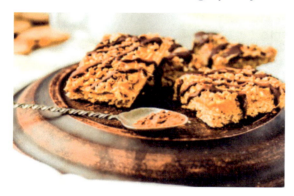

Ingredients:
- 150 g rolled oats
- 50 g shredded coconut
- 50 g dark chocolate chips
- 50 ml coconut oil, melted
- 30 ml maple syrup

Instructions:
1. Combine oats, shredded coconut, chocolate chips, melted coconut oil, and maple syrup in a mixing bowl. Mix well.
2. Press the mixture into a lined baking dish.
3. Chill in the refrigerator for 1 hour or until firm.
4. Cut into bars and serve.

Nutritional information: 210 calories, 3 g protein, 20 g carbohydrates, 12 g fat, 3 g fiber, 0 mg cholesterol, 20 mg sodium, 150 mg potassium.

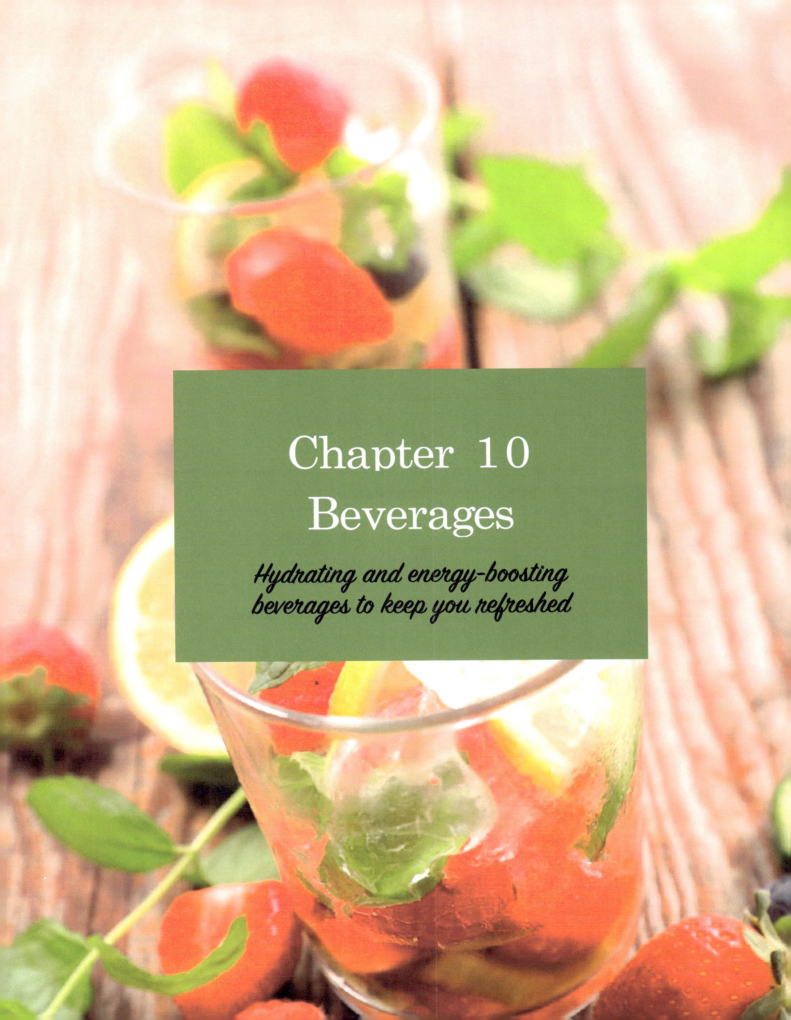

Chapter 10
Beverages

Hydrating and energy-boosting beverages to keep you refreshed

Green Energy Booster Smoothie

Yield: 2 servings | Prep time: 5 minutes | Cook time: 0 minutes

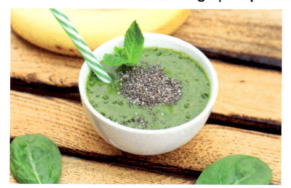

Ingredients:
- 250 ml almond milk (unsweetened)
- 100 g baby spinach
- 1 medium banana (120 g)
- 150 g frozen pineapple chunks
- 1 tbsp chia seeds (10 g)
- 1 tbsp almond butter (15 g)
- 1 tsp spirulina powder (5 g, optional)

Instructions:
1. Add almond milk, baby spinach, banana, frozen pineapple, chia seeds, almond butter, and spirulina powder (if using) to a blender.
2. Blend until smooth and creamy.
3. Pour into two glasses and serve immediately.

Nutritional information: 220 calories, 6 g protein, 35 g carbohydrates, 8 g fat, 7 g fiber, 0 mg cholesterol, 110 mg sodium, 520 mg potassium.

Citrus Hydration Elixir

Yield: 2 servings | Prep time: 5 minutes | Cook time: 0 minutes

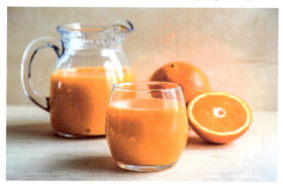

Ingredients:
- 500 ml coconut water
- 100 ml orange juice (freshly squeezed)
- 50 ml lime juice (freshly squeezed)
- 1 tbsp honey (optional, 15 g)
- 4-6 mint leaves
- Ice cubes (optional)

Instructions:
1. Combine coconut water, orange juice, lime juice, and honey in a large pitcher.
2. Stir well to dissolve the honey.
3. Pour into glasses over ice and garnish with mint leaves.

Nutritional information: 85 calories, 1 g protein, 20 g carbohydrates, 0 g fat, 1 g fiber, 0 mg cholesterol, 80 mg sodium, 470 mg potassium.

Golden Turmeric Latte with Coconut Milk

Yield: 2 servings | Prep time: 5 minutes | Cook time: 5 minutes

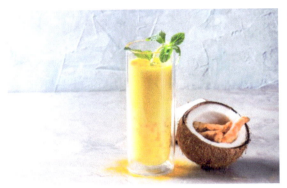

Ingredients:
- 500 ml coconut milk (unsweetened)
- 1 tsp ground turmeric (5 g)
- 1 tsp ground cinnamon (5 g)
- 1 tbsp maple syrup (15 g)
- 1/2 tsp ground ginger (2.5 g)
- Pinch of black pepper

Instructions:
1. Heat coconut milk over medium heat in a small saucepan until warm (do not boil).
2. Whisk in turmeric, cinnamon, ginger, black pepper, and maple syrup.
3. Pour into mugs and serve warm.

Nutritional information: 150 calories, 1 g protein, 10 g carbohydrates, 14 g fat, 1 g fiber, 0 mg cholesterol, 10 mg sodium, 150 mg potassium.

Berry-Chia Antioxidant Refresher

Yield: 2 servings | Prep time: 5 minutes | Cook time: 0 minutes

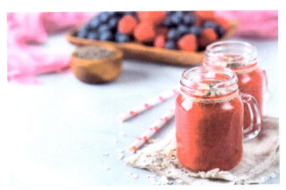

Ingredients:
- 250 ml water
- 150 g mixed berries (blueberries, raspberries, and strawberries)
- 1 tbsp chia seeds (10 g)
- 1 tbsp honey (optional, 15 g)
- Ice cubes (optional)

Instructions:
1. Blend water, mixed berries, and honey until smooth.
2. Stir in chia seeds and let sit for 5 minutes to thicken slightly.
3. Pour into glasses over ice if desired, and serve.

Nutritional information: 90 calories, 1 g protein, 18 g carbohydrates, 2 g fat, 6 g fiber, 0 mg cholesterol, 5 mg sodium, 180 mg potassium.

Zesty Ginger-Lemon Vitality Tonic

Yield: 2 servings | Prep time: 5 minutes | Cook time: 0 minutes

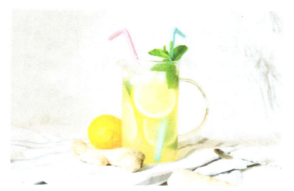

Ingredients:
- 5500 ml water
- 1 tbsp freshly grated ginger (15 g)
- 50 ml lemon juice (freshly squeezed)
- 1 tbsp honey (optional, 15 g)
- Ice cubes (optional)

Instructions:
1. Combine water, grated ginger, lemon juice, and honey in a pitcher.
2. Stir well and strain into glasses over ice.

Nutritional information: 30 calories, 0 g protein, 7 g carbohydrates, 0 g fat, 0 g fiber, 0 mg cholesterol, 5 mg sodium, 50 mg potassium.

Minty Matcha Iced Tea

Yield: 2 servings | Prep time: 5 minutes | Cook time: 0 minutes

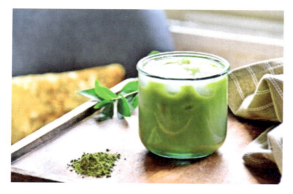

Ingredients:
- 250 ml water (hot, 80°C)
- 1 tsp matcha powder (2 g)
- 4-6 fresh mint leaves
- 1 tbsp honey (optional, 15 g)
- 150 ml cold water
- Ice cubes

Instructions:
1. Whisk matcha powder into hot water until smooth.
2. Add honey (if using) and stir until dissolved.
3. Combine matcha mixture, cold water, and mint leaves in a pitcher.
4. Serve over ice in glasses.

Nutritional information: 30 calories, 0 g protein, 8 g carbohydrates, 0 g fat, 0 g fiber, 0 mg cholesterol, 0 mg sodium, 40 mg potassium.

Revitalizing Watermelon Cucumber Cooler

Yield: 2 servings | Prep time: 5 minutes | Cook time: 0 minutes

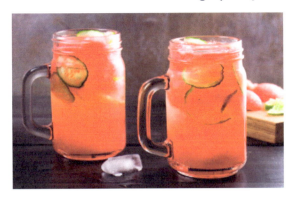

Ingredients:
- 300 g watermelon (seedless, cubed)
- 150 g cucumber (peeled and chopped)
- 1 tbsp lime juice (15 ml)
- 1 tsp honey (optional, 5 g)
- Ice cubes

Instructions:
1. Blend watermelon, cucumber, lime juice, and honey until smooth.
2. Strain through a fine sieve if desired.
3. Pour over ice and serve.

Nutritional information: 60 calories, 1 g protein, 15 g carbohydrates, 0 g fat, 1 g fiber, 0 mg cholesterol, 5 mg sodium, 180 mg potassium.

Spiced Apple Cinnamon Energy Infusion

Yield: 2 servings | Prep time: 5 minutes | Cook time: 10 minutes

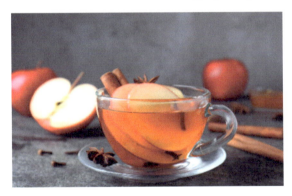

Ingredients:
- 500 ml water
- 1 medium apple (150 g, sliced)
- 1 cinnamon stick
- 1 tbsp honey (optional, 15 g)

Instructions:
1. Combine water, apple slices, and cinnamon sticks in a small saucepan.
2. Bring to a simmer over medium heat and cook for 10 minutes.
3. Strain into mugs, stir in honey if desired, and serve warm.

Nutritional information: 50 calories, 0 g protein, 13 g carbohydrates, 0 g fat, 2 g fiber, 0 mg cholesterol, 5 mg sodium, 100 mg potassium.

Creamy Avocado-Banana Power Shake

Yield: 2 servings | Prep time: 5 minutes | Cook time: 0 minutes

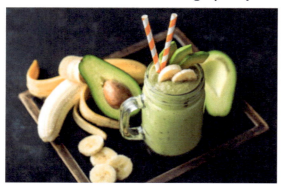

Ingredients:
- 250 ml almond milk (unsweetened)
- 1 medium banana (120 g)
- 1/2 medium avocado (75 g)
- 1 tbsp honey (optional, 15 g)
- 1 tsp vanilla extract (5 ml)
- Ice cubes

Instructions:
1. Blend almond milk, banana, avocado, honey, and vanilla extract until smooth and creamy.
2. Pour into glasses and serve immediately.

Nutritional information: 240 calories, 3 g protein, 29 g carbohydrates, 12 g fat, 6 g fiber, 0 mg cholesterol, 50 mg sodium, 400 mg potassium.

Pineapple-Mango Electrolyte Smoothie

Yield: 2 servings | Prep time: 5 minutes | Cook time: 0 minutes

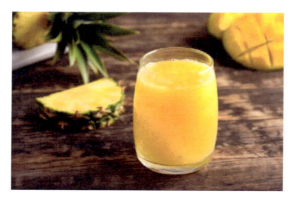

Ingredients:
- 200 g frozen pineapple chunks
- 150 g frozen mango chunks
- 250 ml coconut water
- 1 tsp lime juice (5 ml)
- 1 tbsp honey (optional, 15 g)

Instructions:
1. Blend pineapple, mango, coconut water, lime juice, and honey until smooth.
2. Pour into glasses and serve immediately.

Nutritional information: 140 calories, 1 g protein, 35 g carbohydrates, 0 g fat, 2 g fiber, 0 mg cholesterol, 80 mg sodium, 350 mg potassium.

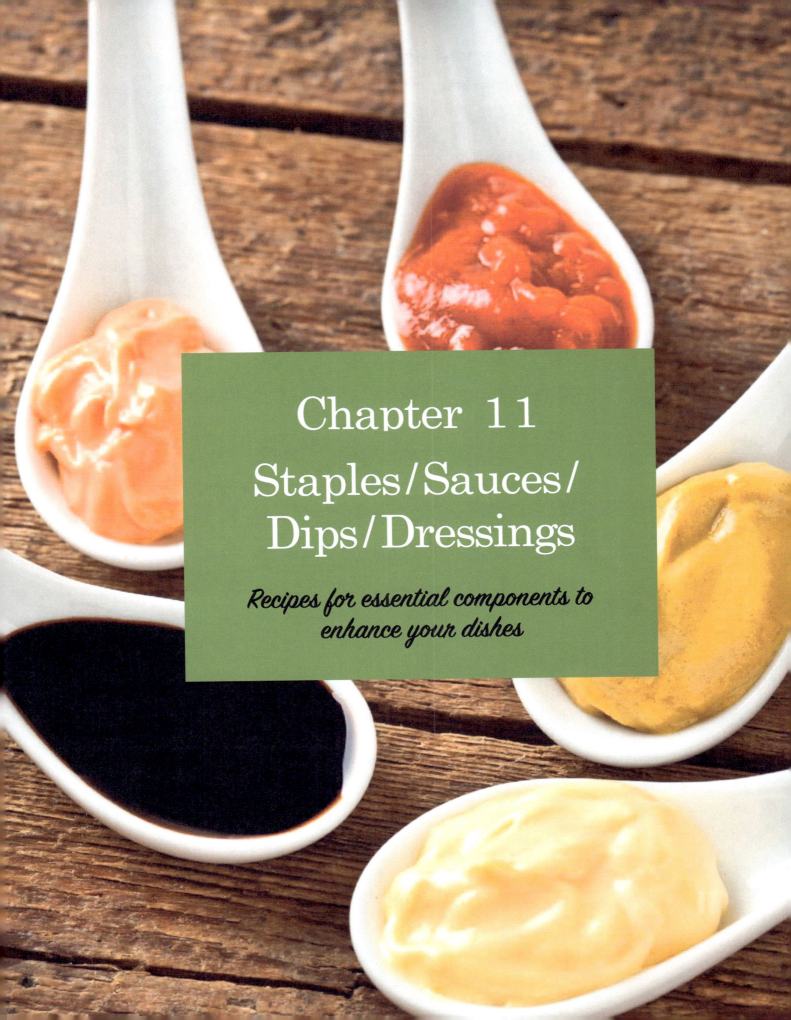

Chapter 11

Staples/Sauces/Dips/Dressings

Recipes for essential components to enhance your dishes

Creamy Avocado Lime Dressing

Yield: 4 servings | Prep time: 10 minutes | Cook time: 0 minutes

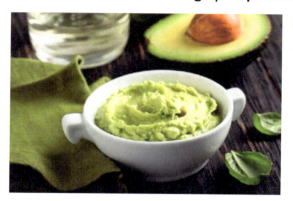

Ingredients:

- 2 ripe avocados (about 250 g)
- 60 ml fresh lime juice
- 60 ml olive oil
- 60 ml water (adjust for desired consistency)
- 2 garlic cloves, minced
- 5 g fresh cilantro, chopped
- 2 g ground cumin
- 1 g sea salt

Instructions:

1. Scoop out the avocado flesh and place it in a blender.
2. Add lime juice, olive oil, water, garlic, cilantro, cumin, and salt.
3. Blend until smooth, adding more water if needed to achieve desired consistency.
4. Serve immediately or store in an airtight container in the fridge for up to 3 days.

Nutritional information: 190 calories, 2 g protein, 5 g carbohydrates, 18 g fat, 3 g fiber, 0 mg cholesterol, 180 mg sodium, 345 mg potassium.

Zesty Lemon Tahini Sauce

Yield: 4 servings | Prep time: 5 minutes | Cook time: 0 minutes

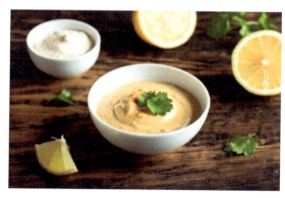

Ingredients:

- 120 g tahini
- 60 ml fresh lemon juice
- 60 ml water
- 1 garlic clove, minced
- 5 g fresh parsley, chopped (optional)
- 1 g sea salt

Instructions:

1. Combine tahini, lemon juice, water, garlic, and salt in a bowl.
2. Whisk until smooth and creamy, adding more water if needed.
3. Stir in parsley if using.
4. Serve immediately or store in the refrigerator for up to 1 week.

Nutritional information: 140 calories, 4 g protein, 5 g carbohydrates, 12 g fat, 2 g fiber, 0 mg cholesterol, 80 mg sodium, 60 mg potassium.

Herbed Olive Oil Vinaigrette

Yield: 4 servings | Prep time: 5 minutes | Cook time: 0 minutes

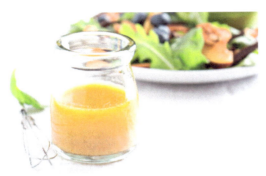

Ingredients:
- 60 ml extra virgin olive oil
- 30 ml red wine vinegar
- 5 g Dijon mustard
- 5 g fresh basil, chopped
- 2 g dried oregano
- 1 garlic clove, minced
- 1 g sea salt

Instructions:
1. Combine olive oil, vinegar, mustard, basil, oregano, garlic, and salt in a jar.
2. Shake well until emulsified.
3. Use immediately or store in the refrigerator for up to 1 week.

Nutritional information: 110 calories, 0 g protein, 1 g carbohydrates, 12 g fat, 0 g fiber, 0 mg cholesterol, 55 mg sodium, 5 mg potassium.

Spicy Roasted Red Pepper Hummus

Yield: 4 servings | Prep time: 10 minutes | Cook time: 0 minutes

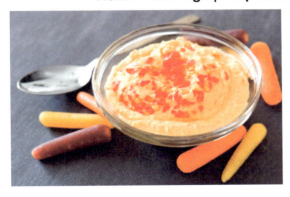

Ingredients:
- 400 g canned chickpeas, drained and rinsed
- 100 g roasted red peppers
- 30 ml fresh lemon juice
- 30 g tahini
- 10 ml olive oil
- 1 garlic clove, minced
- 2 g smoked paprika
- 1 g cayenne pepper
- 1 g sea salt

Instructions:
1. Combine all ingredients in a food processor.
2. Blend until smooth, adding a tablespoon of water if needed for consistency.
3. Serve chilled or at room temperature.

Nutritional information: 160 calories, 6 g protein, 19 g carbohydrates, 7 g fat, 5 g fiber, 0 mg cholesterol, 170 mg sodium, 200 mg potassium.

Classic Cashew Cream Sauce

Yield: 4 servings | Prep time: 10 minutes (plus soaking) | Cook time: 0 minutes

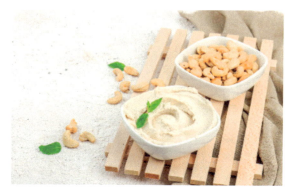

Ingredients:
- 150 g raw cashews (soaked for 2 hours, drained)
- 120 ml water
- 15 ml lemon juice
- 2 g garlic powder
- 1 g sea salt

Instructions:
1. Blend soaked cashews with water, lemon juice, garlic powder, and salt until smooth.
2. Adjust seasoning or add more water if needed for desired consistency.
3. Use immediately or refrigerate for up to 5 days.

Nutritional information: 180 calories, 5 g protein, 10 g carbohydrates, 14 g fat, 1 g fiber, 0 mg cholesterol, 60 mg sodium, 150 mg potassium.

Rich Sun-Dried Tomato Pesto

Yield: 4 servings | Prep time: 10 minutes | Cook time: 0 minutes

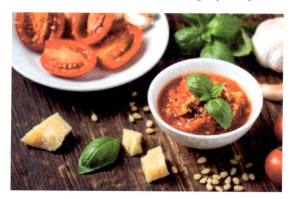

Ingredients:
- 100 g sun-dried tomatoes (packed in oil, drained)
- 30 g pine nuts
- 30 g grated Parmesan cheese
- 2 garlic cloves, minced
- 60 ml olive oil
- 5 g fresh basil leaves
- 1 g sea salt

Instructions:
1. Combine sun-dried tomatoes, pine nuts, Parmesan, garlic, olive oil, basil, and salt in a food processor.
2. Blend until smooth, scraping down the sides as needed.
3. Serve immediately or store in an airtight container in the refrigerator for up to 1 week.

Nutritional information: 200 calories, 4 g protein, 5 g carbohydrates, 18 g fat, 1 g fiber, 5 mg cholesterol, 150 mg sodium, 150 mg potassium.

Refreshing Cucumber Yogurt Dip

Yield: 4 servings | Prep time: 5 minutes | Cook time: 0 minutes

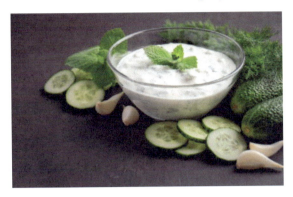

Ingredients:
- 200 g plain Greek yogurt
- 100 g cucumber, grated and drained
- 5 g fresh dill, chopped
- 5 g fresh mint, chopped
- 1 garlic clove, minced
- 5 ml fresh lemon juice
- 1 g sea salt

Instructions:
1. Combine yogurt, cucumber, dill, mint, garlic, lemon juice, and salt in a bowl.
2. Stir until well mixed.
3. Serve chilled or store in the refrigerator for up to 3 days.

Nutritional information: 60 calories, 5 g protein, 3 g carbohydrates, 2 g fat, 0 g fiber, 5 mg cholesterol, 50 mg sodium, 100 mg potassium.

Homemade Golden Turmeric Mustard

Yield: 4 servings | Prep time: 5 minutes | Cook time: 5 minutes

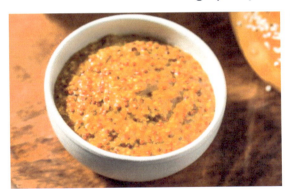

Ingredients:
- 0 g yellow mustard seeds
- 60 ml apple cider vinegar
- 30 ml water
- 2 g ground turmeric
- 1 g sea salt

Instructions:
1. Combine mustard seeds, vinegar, water, turmeric, and salt in a saucepan.
2. Simmer on low heat for 5 minutes.
3. Allow the mixture to cool, then blend to the desired consistency.
4. Store in a sterilized jar in the refrigerator for up to 1 month.

Nutritional information: 20 calories, 1 g protein, 2 g carbohydrates, 1 g fat, 1 g fiber, 0 mg cholesterol, 50 mg sodium, 20 mg potassium.

Sweet and Tangy Maple Balsamic Glaze

Yield: 4 servings | Prep time: 2 minutes | Cook time: 8 minutes

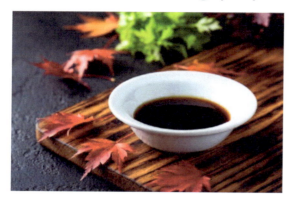

Ingredients:
- 60 ml balsamic vinegar
- 15 ml maple syrup

Instructions:
1. Combine balsamic vinegar and maple syrup in a small saucepan.
2. Simmer over low heat for 8 minutes, stirring occasionally, until thickened.
3. Let cool and drizzle over salads or roasted vegetables.

Nutritional information: 50 calories, 0 g protein, 11 g carbohydrates, 0 g fat, 0 g fiber, 0 mg cholesterol, 5 mg sodium, 40 mg potassium.

Simple Garlic Herb Butter Spread

Yield: 4 servings | Prep time: 5 minutes | Cook time: 0 minutes

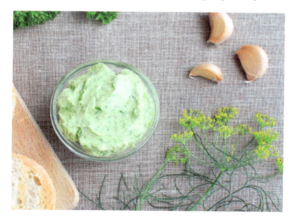

Ingredients:
- 100 g unsalted butter, softened
- 2 garlic cloves, minced
- 5 g fresh parsley, chopped
- 2 g dried thyme
- 1 g sea salt

Instructions:
1. Combine softened butter, garlic, parsley, thyme, and salt in a bowl.
2. Mix well until evenly combined.
3. Store in an airtight container in the refrigerator for up to 1 week.

Nutritional information: 90 calories, 0 g protein, 0 g carbohydrates, 10 g fat, 0 g fiber, 25 mg cholesterol, 40 mg sodium, 5 mg potassium.

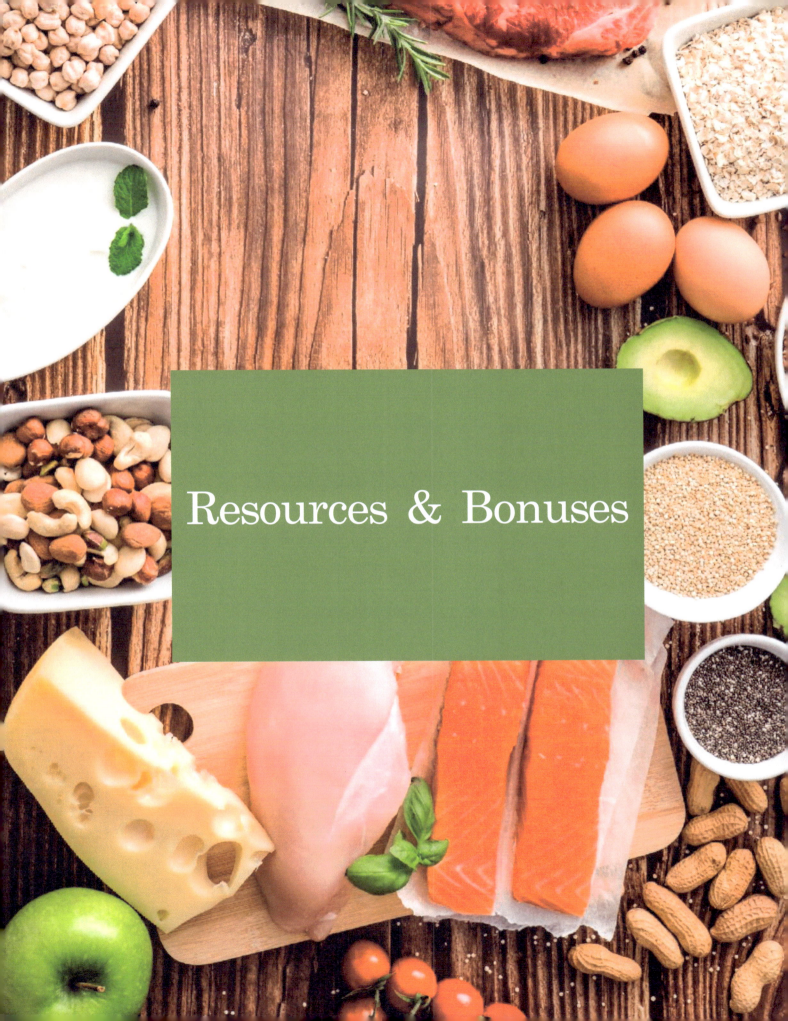

Resources & Bonuses

Ingredient Substitutions

If you're missing an ingredient or need to adjust for dietary preferences, these substitutions will help you maintain flavor and nutrition in your meals.

Grains and Carbs

- **Quinoa**: Swap with bulgur, farro, or millet for a similar texture and nutrient profile.
- **Brown Rice**: Replace with wild rice, barley, or cauliflower rice for a low-carb option.

Proteins

- **Chicken or Turkey**: Substitute with tofu, tempeh, or jackfruit for a plant-based alternative.
- **Eggs (for baking)**: Use flaxseed meal (1 tablespoon flaxseed + 3 tablespoons water = 1 egg) or unsweetened applesauce.

Dairy

- **Milk**: Replace with almond, oat, or coconut milk.
- **Butter**: Use coconut oil, avocado, or plant-based spreads.

Sweeteners

- **Sugar**: Substitute with honey, maple syrup, or stevia, adjusting quantities for sweetness.
- **Honey (for vegans)**: Use agave syrup or date syrup.

Thickeners

- **Flour**: Swap with arrowroot powder, cornstarch, or almond flour for gluten-free options.

Tips for Maximizing Your Resources

1. Create a Kitchen Essentials Kit

Stock your pantry with staples like whole grains, legumes, olive oil, spices, and nuts for quick, versatile meals.

2. Learn Basic Knife Skills

Invest in a good-quality chef's knife and practice chopping techniques to save time and effort in the kitchen.

3. Use Technology to Streamline Cooking

Smart devices like digital scales, blenders, and instant pots can simplify meal prep and ensure precision.

4. Batch Prep for Busy Days

Double recipes and freeze portions for convenient, healthy meals during hectic weeks.

Exclusive Bonus Material
30-Day Good Energy Meal Plan

This plan includes three balanced meals and two optional snacks per day to meet your nutritional needs and support metabolic health. Recipes are chosen for their simplicity, flavor, and alignment with proven dietary science.

Key Features:

- **Energy-Focused Breakfasts**: Whole grains, healthy fats, and lean proteins to sustain energy all morning.
- **Nourishing Lunches**: Fiber-packed vegetables, energizing proteins, and complex carbs for midday fuel.
- **Satisfying Dinners**: Balanced, light dishes designed to support digestion and end the day on a healthy note.
- **Optional Snacks**: Wholesome options to curb cravings and stabilize energy levels.
-

30-Day Good Energy Meal Plan

Day	Breakfast	Lunch	Dinner	Snack
1	Berry Bliss Overnight Oats with Almond Butter	Creamy Roasted Tomato Basil Soup	Lemon Herb Salmon with Quinoa Salad	Crunchy Chickpea Snack Bites
2	Power-Up Green Smoothie with Spinach and Mango	Mediterranean Chickpea Salad with Lemon-Tahini Dressing	Grilled Flank Steak with Chimichurri Sauce	Dark Chocolate Avocado Mousse
3	Protein-Packed Breakfast Burrito with Black Beans	Golden Turmeric and Ginger Carrot Soup	Garlic Honey Glazed Chicken Thighs	Sweet Potato Brownies
4	Fluffy Egg White and Veggie Omelette	Asian-Inspired Cabbage Slaw with Sesame-Ginger Dressing	Slow-roasted lamb Shanks in Red Wine Sauce	Minty Matcha Iced Tea
5	Warm Apple-Cinnamon Quinoa Bowl	Classic Shepherd's Pie with Ground Lamb	Sweet and Savory Pork Stir-Fry with Pineapple	Peanut Butter Banana Protein Muffins
6	Avocado and Smoked Salmon Toast	Rainbow Veggie Salad with Creamy Yogurt Dill Dressing	Spicy Tuna Poke Bowl with Avocado	Greek-Style Stuffed Grape Leaves with Lemon Sauce
7	Energy-Boosting Peanut Butter Banana Smoothie	Mediterranean Orzo Salad with Olives and Feta	Garlic Butter Shrimp with Zucchini Noodles	Oatmeal Energy Cookies with Almond Butter
8	Chia Seed Pudding with Fresh Berries	Broccoli and Cashew Stir-Fry with Ginger Soy Sauce	Honey Garlic Glazed Pork Chops	Spiced Apple Cinnamon Energy Infusion
9	Sweet Potato and Chickpea Breakfast Bowl	Hearty Lentil and Vegetable Stew	Classic Chicken and Quinoa Soup	Baked Zucchini Chips with Lemon-Herb Dip
10	Zucchini and Feta Muffins	Mediterranean Chickpea and Spinach Soup	Crispy Baked Cod with Sweet Potato Wedges	Wholesome Trail Mix Energy Clusters
11	Lemon Blueberry Greek Yogurt Bars	Protein-Packed Lentil and Arugula Salad with Honey-Mustard Dressing	Grilled Eggplant with Garlic Yogurt Sauce	Zesty Ginger-Lemon Vitality Tonic
12	Golden Turmeric Latte with Coconut Milk	Creamy Tomato and Basil Risotto	Spicy Grilled Chicken with Cilantro Lime Sauce	Sweet and Tangy Maple Balsamic Glaze
13	Matcha Green Tea Bliss Balls	Roasted Beet and Arugula Salad with Citrus Dressing	Tender Pulled Pork with Smoky Barbecue Sauce	Oven-Roasted Garlic Parmesan Cauliflower
14	Quinoa Chocolate Chip Protein Bites	Mediterranean-Style Hummus Platter with Veggie Sticks	Lemon Dill Fish Soup	Dark Chocolate Avocado Truffles

Day	Breakfast	Lunch	Dinner	Snack
15	Peanut Butter Banana Smoothie	Crispy Kale Caesar Salad with a Twist of Garlic	Mediterranean Grilled Lamb Kebabs with Tzatziki Sauce	Sweet Potato Wedges with Spicy Yogurt Dip
16	Fluffy Egg White and Veggie Omelette	Classic Chicken and Vegetable Stir-Fry	Slow-Roasted Lamb Shanks in Red Wine Sauce	Herbed Quinoa-Stuffed Bell Peppers
17	Coconut Chia Pudding with Fresh Berries	Savory Sweet Potato and Coconut Curry Stew	Maple-Glazed Turkey Tenderloins with Garlic Mashed Potatoes	Apple Cinnamon Crumble with Oat Topping
18	Creamy Avocado-Banana Power Shake	Watermelon and Feta Salad with Mint and Balsamic Drizzle	Classic Mussels in White Wine Sauce	Lentil and Spinach Energy Balls
19	Sweet Potato and Kale Hash with a Poached Egg	Mediterranean Chickpea Salad with Lemon-Tahini Dressing	Herbed Pork Tenderloin with Roasted Vegetables	Spicy Roasted Red Pepper Hummus
20	Green Energy Booster Smoothie	Broccoli and Cashew Stir-Fry with Ginger Soy Sauce	Crispy Garlic and Rosemary Pork Cutlets	Roasted Beet and Goat Cheese Salad Cups
21	Warm Apple-Cinnamon Quinoa Bowl	Grilled Eggplant with Garlic Yogurt Sauce	Lobster Tails with Lemon Herb Butter	Mushroom and Herb Polenta Bites
22	Avocado and Smoked Salmon Toast	Classic Chicken and Vegetable Stir-Fry	Baked Spinach and Feta Stuffed Portobello Mushrooms	Minty Matcha Iced Tea
23	Berry Bliss Overnight Oats with Almond Butter	Zesty Quinoa and Avocado Salad with Lime Vinaigrette	Scallop and Mango Ceviche	Crunchy Chickpea Snack Bites
24	Energy-Boosting Peanut Butter Banana Smoothie	Sweet Potato and Chickpea Breakfast Bowl	Grilled Flank Steak with Chimichurri Sauce	Peanut Butter Banana Protein Muffins
25	Chia Seed Pudding with Fresh Berries	Mediterranean Chickpea and Spinach Soup	Sweet and Savory Pork Stir-Fry with Pineapple	Zesty Ginger-Lemon Vitality Tonic
26	Golden Turmeric Latte with Coconut Milk	Protein-Packed Lentil and Arugula Salad with Honey-Mustard Dressing	Crispy Baked Cod with Sweet Potato Wedges	Dark Chocolate Avocado Truffles
27	Lemon Blueberry Greek Yogurt Bars	Mediterranean-Style Hummus Platter with Veggie Sticks	Mediterranean Grilled Lamb Kebabs with Tzatziki Sauce	Sweet Potato Wedges with Spicy Yogurt Dip
28	Coconut Chia Pudding with Fresh Berries	Savory Sweet Potato and Coconut Curry Stew	Maple-Glazed Turkey Tenderloins with Garlic Mashed Potatoes	Apple Cinnamon Crumble with Oat Topping
29	Fluffy Egg White and Veggie Omelette	Classic Chicken and Vegetable Stir-Fry	Slow-Roasted Lamb Shanks in Red Wine Sauce	Herbed Quinoa-Stuffed Bell Peppers
30	Green Energy Booster Smoothie	Watermelon and Feta Salad with Mint and Balsamic Drizzle	Lobster Tails with Lemon Herb Butter	Mushroom and Herb Polenta Bites

Printable Shopping List Templates

Table 1: Fresh Produce

Category	Items
Fruits	Apples, bananas, mangoes, avocados, berries (blueberries, strawberries, raspberries), lemons, limes
Vegetables	Spinach, kale, zucchini, sweet potatoes, carrots, onions, tomatoes, bell peppers, cucumbers
Herbs	Basil, parsley, cilantro, dill, rosemary, thyme, mint
Root Veggies	Potatoes, parsnips, turnips, beets

Table 2: Proteins

Category	Items
Meats	Chicken breasts, turkey cutlets, beef tenderloin, ground lamb, pork chops, lamb shanks
Seafood	Salmon, shrimp, cod, mussels, lobster tails, scallops
Plant-Based	Black beans, chickpeas, lentils, quinoa, tofu
Eggs & Dairy	Eggs, egg whites, Greek yogurt, feta cheese, almond milk

Table 3: Grains & Pantry Staples

Category	Items
Grains	Rolled oats, quinoa, barley, whole-wheat pasta, orzo
Pantry Staples	Olive oil, coconut oil, vegetable stock, balsamic vinegar, tahini, peanut butter, almond butter
Canned Goods	Canned tomatoes, chickpeas, coconut milk

Table 4: Spices & Sweeteners

Category	Items
Spices	Turmeric, cinnamon, paprika, garlic powder, chili flakes, ginger
Sweeteners	Honey, maple syrup, vanilla extract

Table 5: Baking & Snacks

Category	Items
Baking Staples	Almond flour, baking powder, cocoa powder
Snacks	Almonds, cashews, dark chocolate, nutritional yeast, trail mix ingredients

Table 6: Sauces & Condiments

Category	Items
Sauces	Cashew cream sauce, pesto, mustard
Dips & Spreads	Hummus, Greek yogurt-based dips

Table 7: Beverages

Category	Items
Hydration Boosters	Coconut water, sparkling water, cucumber, watermelon
Smoothie Bases	Almond milk, coconut milk, Greek yogurt, matcha powder
Fruits for Drinks	Lemons, limes, oranges, berries (blueberries, strawberries, raspberries)
Spices for Beverages	Ginger, turmeric, cinnamon
Special Ingredients	Chia seeds, honey, maple syrup
Teas	Matcha, green tea, herbal tea

Quick Reference Cooking Times for Beginners

Grains and Legumes

Type/Recipe	Size	Liquid (Ratio)	Time	Frozen	Temperature
Quinoa (Warm Apple-Cinnamon Bowl)	Whole	1:2	15–18 min	No	Medium heat
Barley (Beef and Barley Stew)	Pearled	1:3	30–40 min	No	Medium heat
Lentils (Lentil and Arugula Salad, Lentil Stew)	Whole	1:2	25–30 min	Yes	Simmer
Black Beans (Savory Turkey Chili)	Dried (Soaked)	1:3	60–70 min	Yes	Simmer
Chickpeas (Mediterranean Soup)	Whole, Dried (Soaked)	1:3	60–75 min	Yes	Simmer

Vegetables

Type/Recipe	Size	Liquid	Time	Frozen	Temperature
Sweet Potato (Breakfast Bowl, Wedges, Stew)	Cubed	None (Roast)	20–25 min	Yes	200°C (400°F)
Zucchini (Shrimp Zoodles, Muffins)	Sliced or Shredded	None (Sauté/Bake)	3–5 min (Sauté), 20–25 min (Bake)	No	Medium heat/ 180°C (350°F)
Cauliflower (Roasted, Cauliflower Steaks)	Florets	None (Roast)	20–25 min	Yes	200°C (400°F)
Bell Peppers (Stuffed, Salsa)	Whole (Stuffed)	None (Bake)	25–30 min	No	200°C (400°F)
Spinach (Chickpea Soup, Stir-Fry)	Whole leaves	None (Sauté)	2–3 min	Yes	Medium heat

Seafood and Fish

Type/Recipe	Size	Liquid	Time	Frozen	Temperature
Shrimp (Garlic Butter, Shrimp Salad)	Medium	None (Sauté)	5–7 min	Yes	Medium heat (Sauté)
Salmon (Lemon Herb)	Fillet	None (Bake)	12–15 min	Yes	200°C (400°F)
Cod (Crispy Baked)	Fillet	None (Bake)	10–12 min	Yes	200°C (400°F)
Mussels (Classic in White Wine Sauce)	Whole	None (Steam)	5–7 min	No	High heat (Steam)
Octopus (Mediterranean Grilled)	Whole	1:3 (Boil)	45 min (Tenderize)	Yes	Boil (High heat)

Beef, Pork, and Lamb

Type/Recipe	Size	Liquid	Time	Frozen	Temperature
Beef Tenderloin (Herb-Crusted)	Whole (1 kg)	None (Roast)	20 min/500 g	No	200°C (400°F)
Ground Beef (Shepherd's Pie, Stir-Fry)	500 g portions	None (Sauté)	10–12 min	Yes	Medium heat (Sauté)
Lamb Shanks (Braised in Red Wine)	Whole (Bone-In)	1:2 (Braised)	2–3 hrs	No	Low (Slow cook)
Pork Chops (Honey Garlic Glazed)	Medium cuts	None (Grill)	6–8 min/side	No	Medium-high heat
Pulled Pork (Slow-Cooked)	Whole (Shoulder, 2 kg)	1:2 (Slow cook)	6–8 hrs (Low)	Yes	Low heat (Slow cook)

Poultry and Turkey

Type/Recipe	Size	Liquid	Time	Frozen	Temperature
Chicken Breast (Lemon Herb)	Whole	None (Grill)	6–8 min/side	Yes	Medium-high heat
Chicken Thighs (Garlic Honey Glazed)	Bone-in	None (Bake)	25–30 min	Yes	200°C (400°F)
Turkey Chili (Savory with Black Beans)	Ground turkey + beans	1:3 (Broth/Water)	30–35 min (Simmer)	No	Medium heat
Turkey Meatballs (Herbed in Tomato Sauce)	Small balls	None (Bake)	10–12 min	Yes	200°C (400°F)
Turkey Cutlets (Citrus-Marinated)	Thin slices	None (Sear)	3–5 min/side	Yes	Medium heat

Eggs and Breakfast Staples

Type/Recipe	Size	Liquid	Time	Frozen	Temperature
Egg Whites (Omelette with Veggies)	Whole (Whipped)	None (Sauté)	3–5 min	No	Medium heat (Sauté)
Overnight Oats (Berry Bliss)	Whole	None (Chill)	6–8 hrs (Chill)	No	Refrigerate
Chia Seeds (Pudding)	Whole (Soaked)	None (Chill)	2–4 hrs (Chill)	No	Refrigerate
Sweet Potato (Breakfast Bowl, Hash)	Cubed	None (Roast)	20–25 min	Yes	200°C (400°F)
Zucchini (Muffins)	Shredded	None (Bake)	20–25 min	No	180°C (350°F)

Index of recipes

beef stock
Slow-Cooked Beef and Root Vegetable Stew, 25
Hearty Classic Beef and Barley Stew, 28
Slow-roasted lamb Shanks in Red Wine Sauce, 32
Classic Shepherd's Pie with Ground Lamb, 33
beef tenderloin
Savory Herb-Crusted Beef Tenderloin, 27

beets
Roasted Beet and Arugula Salad with Citrus Dressing, 55
Roasted Beet and Goat Cheese Salad Cups, 64

bell pepper
Classic Chicken and Vegetable Stir-Fry, 37
Quick and Easy Beef Stir-Fry with Vegetables, 27
Sweet and Savory Pork Stir-Fry with Pineapple, 31
Herbed Quinoa-Stuffed Bell Peppers, 60

berries
Berry Bliss Overnight Oats with Almond Butter, 16
Berry-Chia Antioxidant Refresher, 75

black beans
Protein-Packed Breakfast Burrito with Black Beans, 17
Homemade Veggie Burgers with Avocado Spread, 56
Zesty Avocado and Black Bean Salsa, 60

black olives
Mediterranean Orzo Salad with Olives and Feta, 56

bone-in pork chops
Honey Garlic Glazed Pork Chops, 29

breadcrumbs
Savory Herb-Crusted Beef Tenderloin, 27
Crispy Garlic and Rosemary Pork Cutlets, 31
Herbed Turkey Meatballs in Tomato Basil Sauce, 36
Crispy Baked Cod with Sweet Potato Wedges, 42
Baked Spinach and Feta Stuffed Portobello Mushrooms, 53
Homemade Veggie Burgers with Avocado Spread, 56
Baked Zucchini Chips with Lemon-Herb Dip, 63

broccoli florets
Quick and Easy Beef Stir-Fry with Vegetables, 27
Classic Chicken and Vegetable Stir-Fry, 37
Broccoli and Cashew Stir-Fry with Ginger Soy Sauce, 54

brown rice

Spicy Tuna Poke Bowl with Avocado, 42

brown sugar
Vegan Pad Thai with Peanut Sauce, 55

brussels sprouts
Herbed Pork Tenderloin with Roasted Vegetables, 30

butter (or vegan butter)
Classic Shepherd's Pie with Ground Lamb, 33
Mushroom and Herb Polenta Bites, 65
Garlic Butter Shrimp with Zucchini Noodles, 41
Garlic Butter Shrimp with Spinach and Cherry Tomatoes, 43
Maple-glazed turkey Tenderloins with Garlic Mashed Potatoes, 38

butter lettuce leaves
Roasted Beet and Goat Cheese Salad Cups, 64

C
canned black beans
Savory Turkey Chili with Black Beans and Corn, 39

canned chickpeas
Crunchy Chickpea Snack Bites, 59
Mediterranean-Style Hummus Platter with Veggie Sticks, 61
Spicy Roasted Red Pepper Hummus, 81

canned coconut milk
Savory Sweet Potato and Coconut Curry Stew, 24

canned crushed tomatoes
Slow-cooked beef Ragu over Whole-Wheat Pasta, 29
Herbed Turkey Meatballs in Tomato Basil Sauce, 36
Creamy Tomato and Basil Risotto, 53

canned diced tomatoes
Hearty Classic Beef and Barley Stew, 28
Classic Shepherd's Pie with Ground Lamb, 33
Savory Turkey Chili with Black Beans and Corn, 39

carrot
Classic Chicken and Vegetable Stir-Fry, 37
Spicy Tuna Poke Bowl with Avocado, 42
Zesty Lemon and Dill Fish Soup, 25
Hearty Lentil and Vegetable Stew, 22
Golden Turmeric and Ginger Carrot Soup, 23
Classic Chicken and Quinoa Soup, 23
Slow-Cooked Beef and Root Vegetable Stew, 25
Hearty Classic Beef and Barley Stew, 28

Slow-roasted lamb Shanks in Red Wine Sauce, 32
Classic Shepherd's Pie with Ground Lamb, 33
Rainbow Veggie Salad with Creamy Yogurt Dill Dressing, 48
Asian-Inspired Cabbage Slaw with Sesame-Ginger Dressing, 50
Broccoli and Cashew Stir-Fry with Ginger Soy Sauce, 54
Vegan Pad Thai with Peanut Sauce, 55
Homemade Veggie Burgers with Avocado Spread, 56
Quick and Easy Beef Stir-Fry with Vegetables, 27
Mediterranean-Style Hummus Platter with Veggie Sticks, 61

cauliflower
Cauliflower Steaks with Chimichurri Sauce, 57

cauliflower florets
Oven-roasted garlic Parmesan Cauliflower, 62

celery
Hearty Lentil and Vegetable Stew, 22
Mediterranean-Style Hummus Platter with Veggie Sticks, 61
Classic Chicken and Quinoa Soup, 23

celery stalk
Zesty Lemon and Dill Fish Soup, 25
Slow-Cooked Beef and Root Vegetable Stew, 25
Hearty Classic Beef and Barley Stew, 28
Slow-roasted lamb Shanks in Red Wine Sauce, 32

cheddar cheese
Protein-Packed Breakfast Burrito with Black Beans, 17

cherry tomatoes
Lemon Herb Salmon with Quinoa Salad, 41
Garlic Butter Shrimp with Spinach and Cherry Tomatoes, 43
Shrimp and Avocado Salad with Lime Dressing, 45
Zesty Quinoa and Avocado Salad with Lime Vinaigrette, 48
Lentil and Arugula Salad with Honey-Mustard Dressing, 49
Mediterranean Orzo Salad with Olives and Feta, 56
Herbed Quinoa-Stuffed Bell Peppers, 60
Zesty Avocado and Black Bean Salsa, 60
Mediterranean-Style Hummus Platter with Veggie Sticks, 61
Mediterranean Chickpea Salad with Lemon-Tahini Dressing,47

chia seeds

Berry Bliss Overnight Oats with Almond Butter, 16
Power-Up Green Smoothie with Spinach and Mango, 16
Fluffy Egg White and Veggie Omelette, 17
Chia Seed Pudding with Fresh Berries, 19
Coconut Chia Pudding with Fresh Berries, 67
Quinoa Chocolate Chip Protein Bites, 69
Peanut Butter Banana Protein Muffins, 71
Green Energy Booster Smoothie, 74
Berry-Chia Antioxidant Refresher, 75

chicken breast
Hearty Lentil and Vegetable Stew, 22
Classic Chicken and Vegetable Stir-Fry, 37
Lemon Herb Roasted Chicken Breasts, 35
Spicy Grilled Chicken with Cilantro Lime Sauce, 36
Creamy Mushroom and Spinach Stuffed Chicken, 38

chicken broth (low sodium)
Savory Turkey Chili with Black Beans and Corn, 39

chicken stock
Hearty Lentil and Vegetable Stew, 22
Tender Pulled Pork with Smoky Barbecue Sauce, 30

chicken thighs, bone-in, skin-on
Garlic Honey Glazed Chicken Thighs, 35

chickpeas
Sweet Potato and Chickpea Breakfast Bowl, 20
Mediterranean Chickpea and Spinach Soup, 24
Crispy Kale Caesar Salad with a Twist of Garlic, 47
Mediterranean Chickpea Salad with Lemon-Tahini Dressing,47

chopped almonds
Oatmeal Energy Cookies with Almond Butter, 68

cinnamon
Warm Apple-Cinnamon Quinoa Bowl, 18
Oatmeal Energy Cookies with Almond Butter, 68
Apple Cinnamon Crumble with Oat Topping, 70
Peanut Butter Banana Protein Muffins, 71
Golden Turmeric Latte with Coconut Milk, 75

cinnamon stick
Spiced Apple Cinnamon Energy Infusion, 77

cocoa powder
Dark Chocolate Avocado Mousse, 67
Dark Chocolate Avocado Truffle, 71
Sweet Potato Brownies, 72

coconut milk

Sweet Potato and Kale Hash with a Poached Egg, 54
Lemon Blueberry Greek Yogurt Bars, 68
Peanut Butter Banana Protein Muffins, 71

eggplants
Grilled Eggplant with Garlic Yogurt Sauce, 52

F

feta cheese
Sweet Potato and Chickpea Breakfast Bowl, 20
Zucchini and Feta Muffins for On-the-Go Energy, 20
Watermelon and Feta Salad with Mint and Balsamic Drizzle, 49
Baked Spinach and Feta Stuffed Portobello Mushrooms, 53
Herbed Quinoa-Stuffed Bell Peppers, 60
Mediterranean Orzo Salad with Olives and Feta, 56

fish stock
Zesty Lemon and Dill Fish Soup, 25

flank steak
Grilled Flank Steak with Chimichurri Sauce, 28

flaxseed
Energy-Boosting Peanut Butter Banana Smoothie, 19

fresh basil
Herbed Turkey Meatballs in Tomato Basil Sauce, 36
Herbed Olive Oil Vinaigrette, 81
Creamy Tomato and Basil Risotto, 53
Rich Sun-Dried Tomato Pesto, 82

fresh berries
Chia Seed Pudding with Fresh Berries, 19
Coconut Chia Pudding with Fresh Berries, 67

fresh blueberries
Lemon Blueberry Greek Yogurt Bars, 68

fresh cilantro leaves
Grilled Flank Steak with Chimichurri Sauce, 28
Savory Turkey Chili with Black Beans and Corn, 39
Scallop and Mango Ceviche, 45
Zesty Quinoa and Avocado Salad with Lime Vinaigrette, 48
Cauliflower Steaks with Chimichurri Sauce, 57
Zesty Avocado and Black Bean Salsa, 60
Creamy Avocado Lime Dressing, 80
Spicy Grilled Chicken with Cilantro Lime Sauce, 36

fresh dill
Mediterranean Grilled Lamb Kebabs with Tzatziki Sauce, 32
Rainbow Veggie Salad with Creamy Yogurt Dill Dressing, 48
Crispy Zucchini Fritters with Dill Dip, 52
Mini Cucumber and Smoked Salmon Bites, 61
Refreshing Cucumber Yogurt Dip, 83

fresh ginger
Golden Turmeric and Ginger Carrot Soup, 23
Savory Sweet Potato and Coconut Curry Stew, 24
Classic Chicken and Vegetable Stir-Fry, 37
Asian-Inspired Cabbage Slaw with Sesame-Ginger Dressing, 50
Broccoli and Cashew Stir-Fry with Ginger Soy Sauce, 54

fresh lemon juice
Mediterranean Chickpea Salad with Lemon-Tahini Dressing, 47
Spicy Roasted Red Pepper Hummus, 81

fresh lime juice
Creamy Avocado Lime Dressing, 80

fresh mint
Spiced Lamb Kofta with Mint Yogurt Dip, 33
Roasted Beet and Goat Cheese Salad Cups, 64
Refreshing Cucumber Yogurt Dip, 83
Watermelon and Feta Salad with Mint and Balsamic Drizzle, 49
Minty Matcha Iced Tea, 76
Citrus Hydration Elixir, 74

fresh parsley
Grilled Flank Steak with Chimichurri Sauce, 28
Honey Garlic Glazed Pork Chops, 29
Spiced Lamb Kofta with Mint Yogurt Dip, 33
Lemon Herb Roasted Chicken Breasts, 35
Garlic Honey Glazed Chicken Thighs, 35
Herbed Turkey Meatballs in Tomato Basil Sauce, 36
Creamy Mushroom and Spinach Stuffed Chicken, 38
Lemon Herb Salmon with Quinoa Salad, 41
Mediterranean Grilled Octopus with Fresh Herbs, 43
Classic Mussels in White Wine Sauce, 44
Lobster Tails with Lemon Herb Butter, 44
Mediterranean Chickpea Salad with Lemon-Tahini Dressing, 47
Grilled Eggplant with Garlic Yogurt Sauce, 52
Sweet Potato and Kale Hash with a Poached Egg, 54
Mediterranean Orzo Salad with Olives and Feta, 56
Cauliflower Steaks with Chimichurri Sauce, 57

Zesty Lemon Tahini Sauce, 80
Simple Garlic Herb Butter Spread, 84
Baked Zucchini Chips with Lemon-Herb Dip, 63
rice noodles
Vegan Pad Thai with Peanut Sauce, 55

fresh rosemary
Slow-cooked beef Ragu over Whole-Wheat Pasta, 29
Slow-roasted lamb Shanks in Red Wine Sauce, 32
Lemon Herb Roasted Chicken Breasts, 35
Crispy Garlic and Rosemary Pork Cutlets, 31

fresh spinach
Creamy Mushroom and Spinach Stuffed Chicken, 38
Baked Spinach and Feta Stuffed Portobello Mushrooms, 53

fresh thyme leaves
Lemon Herb Roasted Chicken Breasts, 35

frozen mango chunks
Power-Up Green Smoothie with Spinach and Mango, 16
Fluffy Egg White and Veggie Omelette, 17

G

ginger
Quick and Easy Beef Stir-Fry with Vegetables, 27
Golden Turmeric Latte with Coconut Milk, 75
Zesty Ginger-Lemon Vitality Tonic, 76

goat cheese
Roasted Beet and Arugula Salad with Citrus Dressing, 55
Roasted Beet and Goat Cheese Salad Cups, 64
Greek yogurt
Mediterranean Grilled Lamb Kebabs with Tzatziki Sauce, 32
Spiced Lamb Kofta with Mint Yogurt Dip, 33
Crispy Kale Caesar Salad with a Twist of Garlic, 47
Rainbow Veggie Salad with Creamy Yogurt Dill Dressing, 48
Lemon Blueberry Greek Yogurt Bars, 68
Spicy Grilled Chicken with Cilantro Lime Sauce, 36

green cabbage
Asian-Inspired Cabbage Slaw with Sesame-Ginger Dressing, 50

green onion
Spicy Tuna Poke Bowl with Avocado, 42

Asian-Inspired Cabbage Slaw with Sesame-Ginger Dressing, 50
Broccoli and Cashew Stir-Fry with Ginger Soy Sauce, 54
Vegan Pad Thai with Peanut Sauce, 55

ground turmeric
Homemade Golden Turmeric Mustard, 83

H

heavy cream
Creamy Roasted Tomato Basil Soup, 22
Classic Mussels in White Wine Sauce, 44

hoisin sauce
Sweet and Savory Pork Stir-Fry with Pineapple, 31

honey
Oatmeal Energy Cookies with Almond Butter, 68
Energy-Boosting Peanut Butter Banana Smoothie, 19
Honey Garlic Glazed Pork Chops, 29
Garlic Honey Glazed Chicken Thighs, 35
Shrimp and Avocado Salad with Lime Dressing, 45
Lentil and Arugula Salad with Honey-Mustard Dressing, 49
Asian-Inspired Cabbage Slaw with Sesame-Ginger Dressing, 50
Hearty Spinach and Strawberry Salad with Toasted Almonds, 50
Roasted Beet and Arugula Salad with Citrus Dressing, 55
Wholesome Trail Mix Energy Clusters, 65
Lemon Blueberry Greek Yogurt Bars, 68
Lemon Blueberry Greek Yogurt Bars, 68
Quinoa Chocolate Chip Protein Bites, 69
Citrus Hydration Elixir, 74
Zesty Ginger-Lemon Vitality Tonic, 76
Zesty Ginger-Lemon Vitality Tonic, 76
Minty Matcha Iced Tea, 76
Revitalizing Watermelon Cucumber Cooler, 77
Spiced Apple Cinnamon Energy Infusion, 77
Creamy Avocado-Banana Power Shake, 78
Pineapple-Mango Electrolyte Smoothie, 78

hot sauce
Savory Sweet Potato Wedges with Spicy Yogurt Dip, 59

K

Kalamata olives
Mediterranean Chickpea Salad with Lemon-Tahini Dressing, 47

kale

Crispy Kale Caesar Salad with a Twist of Garlic, 47

Sweet Potato and Kale Hash with a Poached Egg, 54

Crispy Kale Chips with Nutritional Yeast, 63

L

lamb

Spiced Lamb Kofta with Mint Yogurt Dip, 33
Classic Shepherd's Pie with Ground Lamb, 33

lamb leg or shoulder

Mediterranean Grilled Lamb Kebabs with Tzatziki Sauce, 32

lamb shanks

Slow-roasted lamb Shanks in Red Wine Sauce, 32

lemon

Avocado and Smoked Salmon Toast, 18
Zesty Lemon and Dill Fish Soup, 25
Lemon Herb Roasted Chicken Breasts, 35
Citrus-Marinated Turkey Cutlets with Roasted Vegetables, 37
Lemon Herb Salmon with Quinoa Salad, 41
Garlic Butter Shrimp with Zucchini Noodles, 41
Mediterranean Grilled Octopus with Fresh Herbs, 43
Lobster Tails with Lemon Herb Butter, 44
Lemon Herb Roasted Chicken Breasts, 35

lemon juice

Mediterranean Grilled Lamb Kebabs with Tzatziki Sauce, 32
Spiced Lamb Kofta with Mint Yogurt Dip, 33
Crispy Kale Caesar Salad with a Twist of Garlic, 47
Rainbow Veggie Salad with Creamy Yogurt Dill Dressing, 48
Grilled Eggplant with Garlic Yogurt Sauce, 52
Roasted Beet and Arugula Salad with Citrus Dressing, 55
Homemade Veggie Burgers with Avocado Spread, 56
Cauliflower Steaks with Chimichurri Sauce, 57
Savory Sweet Potato Wedges with Spicy Yogurt Dip, 59
Mediterranean-Style Hummus Platter with Veggie Sticks, 61
Mini Cucumber and Smoked Salmon Bites, 61
Baked Zucchini Chips with Lemon-Herb Dip, 63
Lemon Blueberry Greek Yogurt Bars, 68
Classic Cashew Cream Sauce, 82

lemon juice (fresh)

Refreshing Cucumber Yogurt Dip, 83
Zesty Ginger-Lemon Vitality Tonic, 76
Zesty Lemon Tahini Sauce, 80

lentil

Lentil and Arugula Salad with Honey-Mustard Dressing, 49
Lentil and Spinach Energy Balls, 62

lime

Power-Up Green Smoothie with Spinach and Mango, 16
Fluffy Egg White and Veggie Omelette, 17
Spicy Grilled Chicken with Cilantro Lime Sauce, 36
Scallop and Mango Ceviche, 45
Shrimp and Avocado Salad with Lime Dressing, 45
Savory Turkey Chili with Black Beans and Corn, 39

lime juice

Zesty Quinoa and Avocado Salad with Lime Vinaigrette, 48
Vegan Pad Thai with Peanut Sauce, 55
Zesty Avocado and Black Bean Salsa, 60
Pineapple-Mango Electrolyte Smoothie, 78
Revitalizing Watermelon Cucumber Cooler, 77

lime juice (fresh)

Citrus Hydration Elixir, 74

lobster tails

Lobster Tails with Lemon Herb Butter, 44

M

mango

Scallop and Mango Ceviche, 45
Pineapple-Mango Electrolyte Smoothie, 78

maple syrup

Warm Apple-Cinnamon Quinoa Bowl, 18
Chia Seed Pudding with Fresh Berries, 19
Maple-glazed turkey Tenderloins with Garlic Mashed Potatoes, 38
Dark Chocolate Avocado Mousse, 67
Coconut Chia Pudding with Fresh Berries, 67
Apple Cinnamon Crumble with Oat Topping, 70
Matcha Green Tea Bliss Balls, 70
Sweet Potato Brownies, 72
Chocolate Coconut Energy Bars, 72
Sweet and Tangy Maple Balsamic Glaze, 84
Berry Bliss Overnight Oats with Almond Butter, 16
Golden Turmeric Latte with Coconut Milk, 75

matcha powder

Matcha Green Tea Bliss Balls, 70

Minty Matcha Iced Tea, 76

milk (or unsweetened plant-based milk)
Classic Shepherd's Pie with Ground Lamb, 33
Maple-glazed turkey Tenderloins with Garlic
Mashed Potatoes, 38

mushrooms
Creamy Mushroom and Spinach Stuffed Chicken,
38
Mushroom and Herb Polenta Bites, 65

mussels
Classic Mussels in White Wine Sauce, 44

N

natural peanut butter
Energy-Boosting Peanut Butter Banana Smoothie,
19

nutritional yeast
Crispy Kale Chips with Nutritional Yeast, 63

O

oats
Berry Bliss Overnight Oats with Almond Butter, 16
Lentil and Spinach Energy Balls, 62
Wholesome Trail Mix Energy Clusters, 65
Oatmeal Energy Cookies with Almond Butter, 68
Lemon Blueberry Greek Yogurt Bars, 68
Quinoa Chocolate Chip Protein Bites, 69
Apple Cinnamon Crumble with Oat Topping, 70
Matcha Green Tea Bliss Balls, 70
Peanut Butter Banana Protein Muffins, 71
Chocolate Coconut Energy Bars, 72

octopus
Mediterranean Grilled Octopus with Fresh Herbs,
43

onion
Golden Turmeric and Ginger Carrot Soup, 23
Savory Sweet Potato and Coconut Curry Stew, 24
Mediterranean Chickpea and Spinach Soup, 24
Slow-Cooked Beef and Root Vegetable Stew, 25
Zesty Lemon and Dill Fish Soup, 25
Hearty Classic Beef and Barley Stew, 28
Slow-cooked beef Ragu over Whole-Wheat Pasta,
29
Slow-roasted lamb Shanks in Red Wine Sauce,
32
Classic Shepherd's Pie with Ground Lamb, 33
Savory Turkey Chili with Black Beans and Corn,
39
Classic Mussels in White Wine Sauce, 44
Creamy Tomato and Basil Risotto, 53

Classic Chicken and Quinoa Soup, 23
Homemade Veggie Burgers with Avocado Spread,
56

orange
Citrus-Marinated Turkey Cutlets with Roasted
Vegetables, 37

orange juice
Roasted Beet and Arugula Salad with Citrus
Dressing, 55

orange juice (fresh)
Citrus Hydration Elixir, 74

orzo pasta
Mediterranean Orzo Salad with Olives and Feta,
56

oyster sauce
Quick and Easy Beef Stir-Fry with Vegetables, 27

P

Parmesan cheese
Savory Herb-Crusted Beef Tenderloin, 27
Creamy Mushroom and Spinach Stuffed Chicken,
38
Crispy Baked Cod with Sweet Potato Wedges, 42
Crispy Kale Caesar Salad with a Twist of Garlic,
47
Creamy Tomato and Basil Risotto, 53
Lentil and Spinach Energy Balls, 62
Baked Zucchini Chips with Lemon-Herb Dip, 63
Rich Sun-Dried Tomato Pesto, 82
Crispy Garlic and Rosemary Pork Cutlets, 31

parsley
Herbed Quinoa-Stuffed Bell Peppers, 60
peanut butter
Vegan Pad Thai with Peanut Sauce, 55
Banana Nice Cream with Peanut Swirl, 69
Peanut Butter Banana Protein Muffins, 71

pearl barley
Hearty Classic Beef and Barley Stew, 28

pine nuts
Rich Sun-Dried Tomato Pesto, 82

pineapple
Sweet and Savory Pork Stir-Fry with Pineapple,
31
Green Energy Booster Smoothie, 74
Pineapple-Mango Electrolyte Smoothie, 78

plain Greek yogurt
Grilled Eggplant with Garlic Yogurt Sauce, 52

Crispy Zucchini Fritters with Dill Dip, 52
Savory Sweet Potato Wedges with Spicy Yogurt Dip, 59
Baked Zucchini Chips with Lemon-Herb Dip, 63
Refreshing Cucumber Yogurt Dip, 83

polenta
Mushroom and Herb Polenta Bites, 65

poppy seeds
Hearty Spinach and Strawberry Salad with Toasted Almonds, 50

pork cutlets
Crispy Garlic and Rosemary Pork Cutlets, 31

pork loin
Sweet and Savory Pork Stir-Fry with Pineapple, 31

pork shoulder
Tender Pulled Pork with Smoky Barbecue Sauce, 30

pork tenderloin
Herbed Pork Tenderloin with Roasted Vegetables, 30

portobello mushrooms
Baked Spinach and Feta Stuffed Portobello Mushrooms, 53

potatoes
Classic Chicken and Quinoa Soup, 23
Slow-Cooked Beef and Root Vegetable Stew, 25
Herbed Pork Tenderloin with Roasted Vegetables, 30
Classic Shepherd's Pie with Ground Lamb, 33
Maple-glazed turkey Tenderloins with Garlic Mashed Potatoes, 38

powdered sugar
Dark Chocolate Avocado Truffle, 71

Q

quinoa
Warm Apple-Cinnamon Quinoa Bowl, 18
Hearty Lentil and Vegetable Stew, 22
Lemon Herb Salmon with Quinoa Salad, 41
Zesty Quinoa and Avocado Salad with Lime Vinaigrette, 48
Herbed Quinoa-Stuffed Bell Peppers, 60
Quinoa Chocolate Chip Protein Bites, 69

R

raw cashews

Classic Cashew Cream Sauce, 82

red bell pepper
Scallop and Mango Ceviche, 45
Mediterranean Chickpea Salad with Lemon-Tahini Dressing,47
Mediterranean-Style Hummus Platter with Veggie Sticks, 61
Rainbow Veggie Salad with Creamy Yogurt Dill Dressing, 48

red cabbage
Rainbow Veggie Salad with Creamy Yogurt Dill Dressing, 48
Asian-Inspired Cabbage Slaw with Sesame-Ginger Dressing, 50

red curry paste
Savory Sweet Potato and Coconut Curry Stew, 24

red onion
Hearty Spinach and Strawberry Salad with Toasted Almonds, 50
Mediterranean Chickpea Salad with Lemon-Tahini Dressing,47
Zesty Quinoa and Avocado Salad with Lime Vinaigrette, 48
Lentil and Arugula Salad with Honey-Mustard Dressing, 49
Lemon Herb Salmon with Quinoa Salad, 41
Scallop and Mango Ceviche, 45
Zesty Avocado and Black Bean Salsa, 60

red peppers
Spicy Roasted Red Pepper Hummus, 81

red wine
Slow-cooked beef Ragu over Whole-Wheat Pasta, 29
Slow-roasted lamb Shanks in Red Wine Sauce, 32

red wine vinegar
Grilled Flank Steak with Chimichurri Sauce, 28
Mediterranean Grilled Octopus with Fresh Herbs, 43
Mediterranean Orzo Salad with Olives and Feta, 56
Cauliflower Steaks with Chimichurri Sauce, 57
Herbed Olive Oil Vinaigrette, 81

rice vinegar
Classic Chicken and Vegetable Stir-Fry, 37
Asian-Inspired Cabbage Slaw with Sesame-Ginger Dressing, 50
Broccoli and Cashew Stir-Fry with Ginger Soy Sauce, 54
roasted peanuts
Vegan Pad Thai with Peanut Sauce, 55

S

salmon fillets
Lemon Herb Salmon with Quinoa Salad, 41

scallops
Scallop and Mango Ceviche, 45

sesame oil
Quick and Easy Beef Stir-Fry with Vegetables, 27
Sweet and Savory Pork Stir-Fry with Pineapple, 31
Classic Chicken and Vegetable Stir-Fry, 37
Asian-Inspired Cabbage Slaw with Sesame-Ginger Dressing, 50
Broccoli and Cashew Stir-Fry with Ginger Soy Sauce, 54
Vegan Pad Thai with Peanut Sauce, 55
Spicy Edamame Pods with Sea Salt and Lime, 64
Spicy Tuna Poke Bowl with Avocado, 42

sesame seeds
Classic Chicken and Vegetable Stir-Fry, 37
Asian-Inspired Cabbage Slaw with Sesame-Ginger Dressing, 50
Spicy Tuna Poke Bowl with Avocado, 42

shredded coconut
Matcha Green Tea Bliss Balls, 70
Dark Chocolate Avocado Truffle, 71
Chocolate Coconut Energy Bars, 72

shrimp
Garlic Butter Shrimp with Zucchini Noodles, 41
Garlic Butter Shrimp with Spinach and Cherry Tomatoes, 43
Shrimp and Avocado Salad with Lime Dressing, 45

smoked salmon
Avocado and Smoked Salmon Toast, 18
Mini Cucumber and Smoked Salmon Bites, 61

snap peas
Sweet and Savory Pork Stir-Fry with Pineapple, 31
Classic Chicken and Vegetable Stir-Fry, 37

soy sauce
Quick and Easy Beef Stir-Fry with Vegetables, 27
Honey Garlic Glazed Pork Chops, 29
Sweet and Savory Pork Stir-Fry with Pineapple, 31
Asian-Inspired Cabbage Slaw with Sesame-Ginger Dressing, 50
Broccoli and Cashew Stir-Fry with Ginger Soy Sauce, 54
Vegan Pad Thai with Peanut Sauce, 55
Spicy Edamame Pods with Sea Salt and Lime, 64
Spicy Tuna Poke Bowl with Avocado, 42

soy sauce low sodium
Garlic Honey Glazed Chicken Thighs, 35
Classic Chicken and Vegetable Stir-Fry, 37

spinach
Power-Up Green Smoothie with Spinach and Mango, 16
Fluffy Egg White and Veggie Omelette, 17
Sweet Potato and Chickpea Breakfast Bowl, 20
Mediterranean Chickpea and Spinach Soup, 24
Garlic Butter Shrimp with Spinach and Cherry Tomatoes, 43
Hearty Spinach and Strawberry Salad with Toasted Almonds, 50
Green Energy Booster Smoothie, 74
Lentil and Spinach Energy Balls, 62

spirulina powder
Green Energy Booster Smoothie, 74

sriracha
Spicy Tuna Poke Bowl with Avocado, 42

strawberries
Hearty Spinach and Strawberry Salad with Toasted Almonds, 50

sun-dried tomatoes
Rich Sun-Dried Tomato Pesto, 82

sunflower seeds
Lentil and Spinach Energy Balls, 62

sweet corn kernels
Savory Turkey Chili with Black Beans and Corn, 39

sweet potatoes
Sweet Potato and Chickpea Breakfast Bowl, 20
Savory Sweet Potato and Coconut Curry Stew, 24
Crispy Baked Cod with Sweet Potato Wedges, 42
Sweet Potato and Kale Hash with a Poached Egg, 54
Savory Sweet Potato Wedges with Spicy Yogurt Dip, 59
Sweet Potato Brownies, 72

T

tahini
Zesty Lemon Tahini Sauce, 80
Classic Cashew Cream Sauce, 82

Y

yellow bell pepper
Mediterranean-Style Hummus Platter with Veggie Sticks, 61
Classic Chicken and Vegetable Stir-Fry, 37

yellow mustard seeds
Homemade Golden Turmeric Mustard, 83

Z

zucchini
Zucchini and Feta Muffins for On-the-Go Energy, 20
Crispy Zucchini Fritters with Dill Dip, 52
Garlic Butter Shrimp with Zucchini Noodles, 41
Baked Zucchini Chips with Lemon-Herb Dip, 63

Thank you for choosing

The Complete Good Energy Cookbook for Beginners

as your companion on the journey to wellness! I hope these recipes have brought simplicity, joy, and nourishment to your table.

If you've found value in these pages and enjoyed the flavorful benefits, I'd love to hear from you!

Your review not only encourages us but also helps others discover the transformative power of balanced, energy-boosting meals. Here's to every bite leading you closer to a healthier, more vibrant life. Thank you for supporting my mission to make wellness achievable for everyone!